"...but there are always miracles."

JACK AND MARY WILLIS

"...but there are

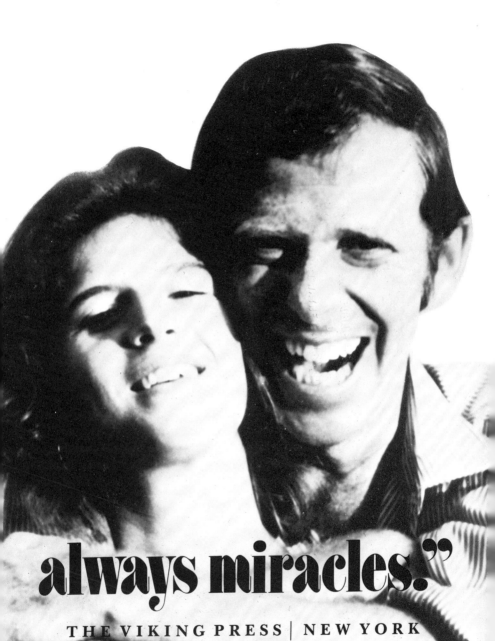

always miracles."

THE VIKING PRESS | NEW YORK

Copyright© 1974 by Jack Willis Productions
All rights reserved
First published in 1974 by The Viking Press, Inc.
625 Madison Avenue, New York, N.Y. 10022
Published simultaneously in Canada by
The Macmillan Company of Canada Limited
SBN 670-19757-2
Library of Congress catalog card number: 73-20946
Printed in U.S.A.
Photograph on title page by Jeff Young

1805921

to joe, janet, and clive

"...but there are always miracles."

jack

I realized I might die, but I wasn't afraid. It seemed painless, even tolerable. I tried to get my legs underneath me, but they wouldn't go. I fought slipping off into unconsciousness. Which way was up? I rolled over and over in the surf, looking for the sunlight through the water. But I couldn't find it, and I was running out of breath. I tried again to get my legs underneath me. They still wouldn't go. I kept rolling and rolling, looking for the light. How long had I been under? It seemed like hours, and I knew I couldn't hold out much longer. What a dumb fucking way to die! I thought, and suddenly my head came free and I yelled for help as loudly as I could.

I felt arms grab me, drag me out of the water along the sandy bottom. I screamed at them to be careful, that I thought I had broken my neck or back. I had no feeling in my body. I was paralyzed from my chest down. They put me on the sand near the edge of the water. Someone brought a piece of driftwood and tucked it under my head. Someone else went to call for help. While we were waiting for the ambulance, the police arrived. They took the log out from under my head and laid me flat on the beach. They asked my name and questioned me about the accident and the lack of feeling and movement in my body. Then, while one went to report in, the other scratched the soles of my feet with a pencil. I could feel it, but it was numb and dull. I felt as if I'd been given a massive dose of Novocain. I could feel pressure but no pain. Most of my body, from the nipples down, was numb.

I tried moving my arms. They seemed all right, although the left one was weak. Mary was kneeling in the sand next to me.

"Move your fingers," she said.

"I can't move them."

"Here. Squeeze my hand," she said, placing her hand in mine.

"I can't," I said. "My fingers are numb. I can't move them. It's as if they were asleep."

"Try your legs."

"I can't. They won't move."

"Try again," she insisted.

I tried. "I can't move anything but my arms."

She looked at me almost in disbelief. Then she reached down, grabbed my legs, and tried to prop them up. They flopped down on the sand.

She looked around as though she expected an answer from the crowd of people that had started to gather. They just stared back. Two ambulance drivers arrived. They also questioned me and tested my feet for feeling. They didn't want to move me until a doctor arrived.

Thoughts came rushing in, confused and uncontrolled. I was happy to be alive. I had fought a terrific battle in the water and had won. But that was over, and now I wanted to go home. Now. But I couldn't. I couldn't move. This couldn't be happening to me. I wanted to go back in time. I wanted another chance. I wanted to undo the moment or redo it differently. TAKE A DIFFERENT WAVE!

I had been body-surfing since I was a kid. I should have known better. I shouldn't have taken that wave. I should have waited for another one, one less dangerous. At least I should have gotten my arms out in front of me. I should have protected my head. It was frightening . . . the one act . . . an accident. I wanted to do it over. I would have done it differently. . . .

All I could see was faces staring at me. I felt like some strange fish that had washed up on the beach, a subject of concern but also of wonderment. I looked at those faces, and tears welled up in my eyes. I may have been touched by their concern, but I may have been crying for myself.

I recognized a familiar feeling. I felt an erection straining against my swimming trunks. At least I could feel that. I looked at Mary. She saw it too, and we smiled. We didn't find out until much later that erections can be signs of severe spinal damage. That is one of the reasons hanging was such a popular spectators' sport: after the victim's neck snapped, he often could be seen, by the bulge in his pants, giving one last salute to life.

Mary got up to talk with the police, and a little blond man with soft hands shielded my eyes from the late-afternoon sun and wiped the sand off my face. He told me not to worry, that I'd be okay. His voice was kind, his hands tender and loving, like a girl's. More tears. I couldn't control them.

I don't remember anything that Mary said to me on the beach that day. I do remember that when I was first pulled out of the water she was nervous, but slowly became calm and comforting, and finally helpful to the police and doctor. We must have said to each other, "Don't worry, it will be all right." We must have said all those things, but I don't remember. It was so unreal. A nightmare.

I again tried to move my right arm and found that I could. I tried my left. It was weaker than the right, but I could move it. I tried my fingers and the rest of my body. I still couldn't make them move. I saw all those people looking at me in a way that I had never been looked at before—as an object of pity.

I remembered once seeing a man pass out in a restaurant. He wasn't drunk, and when he came to, he was embarrassed because his friends insisted on leaving dinner to see him home. Was the embarrassment due to some feeling of inadequacy or to the attention he was getting? I thought how childish he was but felt sure that I'd be the same way in his position. I thought of all that and was surprised that there on the beach I felt no embarrassment at all.

I saw all the concerned faces wanting to help. I could tell they wanted me to move, to jump up and run down the beach as though I'd only had the wind knocked out of me. I could see it in their eyes. What else were they thinking? That it could have been any one of them? Maybe. But serious accidents always seem to happen to the other guy. Somebody else. I'd never really been seriously hurt, even seriously ill. And I hardly knew anyone who had even been in a bad accident, certainly no one who had been paralyzed. I remembered reading about Roy Campanella, who ran his car into a tree and was paralyzed from the neck down. He has to spend the rest of his life in a wheelchair. I was seized with fear . . . a freaky accident, one in a million, and it was happening to me. I didn't want to panic. I didn't want to scare Mary. I tried to tell myself that maybe it wasn't serious. But I knew better. I knew that I was badly hurt. And then I thought, one second I'm healthy, work is challenging, I'm in love; the next second I'm hurt so badly that I might be a basket case for the rest of my life. Maybe I was too secure in my own way. . . . I had it made. Perhaps I could have accepted intellectually that I might be an unfortunate victim of a freak accident, but I couldn't accept it emotionally. These things don't happen to people like me. That's not my destiny. Bullshit.

Contemplate the student at the master's feet on a radiant day when he's feeling wonderful. "Oh, tell me, great master, what is the meaning of life?" The master does not speak but hits the student over the head, breaking his neck and paralyzing him. "That is the meaning of life," he says.

The doctor arrived about fifteen minutes after the ambulance. He was wearing horn-rimmed glasses, and he looked to be in his mid-thirties, about my age. If he'd had a putter in his hand, I wouldn't have been surprised. He was wearing black-and-white cotton checked pants and an open-necked polo shirt. He fit right in with the scene. I thought at first that he was a city doctor whom the hospital had called away from a cocktail party, but I heard an ambulance driver say hello to him, and he told me he was from Southampton and had been called while on late rounds at the hospital.

He walked toward my feet. "Can you feel this?" he said as he scratched my feet just as the ambulance drivers and police had done. He then bent my big toe and asked me what I felt. I told him that he'd bent the toe "up." He then bent it down, and I said, "Down." Then he did the same with my other foot, and I responded correctly. He said that was good, "a very good sign." I didn't ask him why that was a good sign. I just let him work and waited for his diagnosis. Then he asked me to move my arms, which I did, but I couldn't move anything else.

I felt as if I were in a chase in a dream where I'd say, "Move legs," and they wouldn't move. I was making no contact at all with those muscles, no matter how clearly or intensely I willed them to move.

The doctor told me his name was Dr. Spinzia. For some inexplicable reason I couldn't call him Doctor. He was my age, and somehow, in this situation, formality seemed ridiculous. I asked him his first name, and he answered Joe. From then on I called him by his first name.

He cradled my head in his hands while four men lifted me gingerly up onto a board to carry me off the beach to the ambulance. When we got to the sand dunes, Joe lifted my head just a little, and I felt bullets shoot down from my shoulders through my arms into my hands. I felt as though I were being electrocuted. I screamed in pain. Raw nerves were being violated by bone. It was the most intense pain I'd ever felt. I wondered how people withstand torture. I felt the blood go out of my head and thought I might vomit. But as Joe lowered my head a little, the pain ceased. They gently placed me in the ambulance, and then Joe and Mary got in with me. On the way to the hospital Joe kept telling me that he'd seen worse accidents than mine, accidents men had walked away from. Mary asked him what he thought it was. He said it looked like a broken neck and that the vertebrae were pressing against my spine, causing prolonged paralysis.

When we arrived at the hospital, they pushed me right into the X-ray room. I had a weird sensation of dozens of right angles, like a Mondrian gone crazy, and thought that I was facing a glass door or window. Suddenly I had a terrific urge to glance up and catch my own reflection, to see what I looked like. I had the eerie feeling that I was lying on an incline and would be able to see myself in that door or window. I asked Joe. He said I was perfectly horizontal. I was staring at the ceiling.

All of a sudden Joe got excited. "Did you do that?" he asked.

"What?"

"Move your leg."

"No," I said.

"Only reflexes," he muttered as if to himself.

The first X-rays were of my lower back.

"Looks fine so far," Joe said. "Just terrific—no damage, no dislocation, nothing broken."

A few minutes later after more X-rays he said they could find nothing wrong with my neck either. The news seemed good, I thought, but Joe looked troubled.

"What is it?" I said.

"I don't know. I don't know why you're paralyzed if there is no fracture or dislocation. Maybe your spine snapped out of place and back in again, causing serious abrasions. We're just going to have to wait to see what happens. In the meantime," he said, "we're going to put you in traction."

By now I was feeling high from a shot of Demerol. It wasn't like lying on the beach where I had time to think about the consequences of the accident. Now I was involved, even though passively, and wanted to find out what was wrong. The Demerol helped me get outside myself and view all that was happening with a curious kind of objectivity and interest. "Okay," Joe said. "I'm going to drill holes in either side of your head and insert a pair of tongs—they're like ice tongs—into the holes. It won't hurt. You don't have nerves in your skull, and the Novocain will take care of your scalp. Then I'm going to hang weights on you to immobilize your back and neck."

I was wheeled out of X-ray into another room. Joe shaved my head around the ears, and then I felt him make two pencil marks on both sides of my head for the holes. He shot my skull full of Novocain. I looked out of the corner of my eye, expecting to see a high-speed drill. Dismayed, I saw him pick up an old hand drill with what looked like a quarter-inch bit. I braced myself for a shock. I felt the pressure of the drill but felt no pain as it chewed its way into my head. By now the Demerol was really working, and I imagined that my whole being was inside my skull as the drill ripped into me. I could hear the bone being ground, and out of the corner of my eye I could see Joe cranking the drill. He finished one side, then the other. Then with something like toggle bolts he clamped the tongs into my head and suspended big black weights from them. When he finished, two nurses wheeled me down a long hall to a hospital room. All I saw was ceiling.

It had been about three hours since the accident, but time didn't seem to have any shape. I was still in my swimming trunks, still covered with sand. I had no idea whether it was day or night. I felt no pain, and the pull of the weights in my head was strange but not uncomfortable. I still couldn't believe what was happening to me, and I was scared. Mary was waiting for me in my room. She told me that she had called her parents in New York and that they would be out soon. When her parents arrived, I couldn't tell from their eyes how bad off I was. I didn't have to. I knew. We tried to talk, but I drifted off to sleep.

I was awakened by the groans of a man in the bed next to mine. He sounded as if he were in terrible pain. I tried to concentrate on him but couldn't. I realized that there was a nurse with him, and when she saw that I was awake, she came over and cleaned a little of the sand off me. I wondered why they hadn't taken my bathing suit off. She kept calling me chief. "How you doing, chief?" "How'd it happen, chief?" "Hold my hand, chief. Now squeeze my fingers." I tried. I ordered my fingers to move, but nothing happened. I couldn't squeeze her hand, and I felt disappointed that I couldn't. She wiped the sweat off my face and smiled. "Don't get down, chief. Sometimes it takes a while." I tried to smile but couldn't. "Good night, chief," I said, and fell back to sleep.

I hiked up three flights of stairs, Mary opened the door. She was pretty but looked even younger than I had expected. She took my arm while we waited for a taxi. She did it easily, as if we were old friends. My confidence soared out of all proportion to the gesture. It was the tip-off, I said to myself. She likes me. Her simple move established an intimacy and quickly did away with most of the awkwardness of a blind date. And she seemed to be saying that we'd make it.

I don't remember what we talked about, but we talked a lot, not rushed, not manic, but still afraid of pauses. Sometime during dinner I realized I was eating mechanically, shoveling food into my mouth but not tasting. I was working hard to impress her, and if I was at a loss for words and needed time to think, I'd pick up a piece of meat and chew slowly and thoughtfully, buying time for myself. Or if she said something she seemed to think deserved a laugh and I didn't, I would slip her a tight grin that appeared to have great meaning, simply because I'd taken time out from pushing peas onto my fork to grant it. She remembers that after dinner we went for a short walk and that I put my arm around her. Later we went to a bar on the East Side and talked until early morning.

I suppose we talked about all the things people talk about on a first date. She'd been raised in New York and I in Los Angeles. She'd gone to private schools and to Sarah Lawrence, I to public schools and to U.C.L.A. She was a researcher at *Newsweek;* I made documentary films. She was twenty-two and I was thirty-four. She liked older men, and I liked younger women. And we were both Jewish, even though Pleshette sounds French and Willis like a black athlete.

Our second date was on a Sunday afternoon in Central Park. It was late March and the first warm day of the year, the kind of day before the trees begin to blossom, when the earth is still soft and wet, when the sunlight is thin and winter is still present but mixed with the promise of spring. The strollers and children were out sharing the day with kite fliers, athletes, and lovers. We ate hamburgers and hot dogs at the zoo. She looked beautiful to me, slim and young. She talked almost compulsively about herself, the way people who have been terribly lonely and inside themselves for a long time talk. Another neurotic chick, I said to myself, strung-out and unhappy, mixed up about life and love. But it wasn't that way at all. She was simply talking out her own sense of discovery and growth.

I spent most of our third date trying to get her into *her* bed without success and the fourth date trying to get her into *my* bed with success. Apparently it did matter whose bed it was. I was still some kind of intruder in her apartment, that newly found symbol of independence. By summer we were what my Aunt Edith might call "an item."

That summer is only a few years ago, but it seems like twenty. What I remember most clearly is an overwhelming sense of joy and completeness when we were together that got stronger as the year went on. I traveled a lot that summer, working on a new film. I'd return to New York to rich days and joyful nights with Mary. As a child she had precociously shown off for her parents and their friends. Now I was her audience—in the nude, tits bouncing, she'd sing "Ain't She Sweet" and tap-dance a shuffle-off-to-Buffalo into the bathroom. One night she went into the kitchen for a midnight snack of doughnuts and milk and returned wearing only an apron and a bra made out of two doughnuts held together with a ribbon.

That summer we spent long, hot weekends on Long Island. We stayed in a tiny guest house that belonged to an elderly couple and spent days and nights on the beach. We body-surfed together. We began with the tiny waves that break late but roll a long way, high onto the shore. I taught Mary how to get out in front of them, to keep her head up and then ride the wave all the way onto the beach, where we were left covered with sand as the water rolled back to the sea. Then I taught her to go after the big ones, the wave "outside," the wave beyond the others. I showed her how to spot the dangerous ones, the waves that have no water underneath them, that crush down on you or flip you around so that you hit the sand instead of being cushioned on a bed of water. When we saw the right one, we'd run to catch it while it was still swelling. Then we'd swim madly with it, on top and a little out front so that when it crested and broke we would fall what seemed a hundred feet and bounce along toward the shore.

Each time was a first time. No matter how many times we rode the waves, we'd jump up and laugh when it was over and race out, hurdling the tiny waves, diving under the big ones to get out to stand and wait and watch for the one outside.

In *The Magic Mountain* Thomas Mann describes how individual days drag when you are bored but in hindsight seem to have passed quickly because there was a sameness about each of them. And how days that are rich with experience fly by but in retrospect seem to have gone slowly because there is so much to remember. Our days sped by that year. Yet, when we stopped to think about them, it seemed as if time were standing still.

Everyday things took on new meanings. Yet because we were together they became invested with an over-all common meaning. Our concept of time itself changed because we were living to a new and different rhythm. Those tiny boxes of time—eating, sleeping, loving, working, and playing—with which we define our days became blurred around the edges and in the center as well. Eating became a time to share new experiences together and took on a sensuousness of its own. We went to bed to make love and slept only to restore ourselves. Waking in the morning was to make more love. And our work, the days' triumphs and frustrations, added to the whole we shared.

In the fall Mary moved in with me, and neither of us was seeing anyone else. We both thought about marriage but didn't talk about it . . . not until the following spring.

It was a beautiful San Francisco day. We were on the last leg of a month's holiday—three weeks in Mexico, a few days in L.A. with my family, now San Francisco.

We took the cable car to Fisherman's Wharf. I had planned this day to pop the question to Mary. Already drunk with the day and with each other, we had drinks at the Buena Vista, a favorite bar of mine dating back to my basic-training days at Fort Ord when I'd spent my weekends in San Francisco. We walked down to the wharf for a lunch of cracked crab. I tried projecting what I would say and how it would feel to ask Mary to marry me. The problem was that we'd been living together for so long that I didn't know what I should say. It only made me nervous to think ahead, so I decided to say whatever came into my mind at whatever moment I considered appropriate.

I ordered wine and asked that it be brought to the table before lunch, and then, still distracted by what I might say, made small talk. We waited and waited and waited. No wine. I called the waiter and asked again for the wine. He finally brought it along with our lunch. I decided to wait until after lunch when I could order brandy or champagne.

But I felt like a kid on Christmas Eve, who wants to sleep so the night will pass quickly, but who's so excited that he can't and the night seems as if it will never end. Our meal felt that way to me. I couldn't wait any more. I took my wine glass, raised it toward Mary, and tried to catch her eye. I coughed, and she looked up and put some crab in her mouth and waited for me to say something. "I . . ." I began. "Mary . . . will you marry me?" She blushed like a virgin and, still with her mouth full of crab, said, "Yes." We both started laughing, laughing like crazy people, and we both had tears in our eyes.

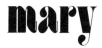

mary

It had been such a perfect day. It felt like the first day of summer—clear blue sky, a hot direct sun, so hot that you could actually feel your already tan skin burn. And the waves were perfect for body-surfing. Jack and I arrived at the beach at eleven thirty and, looking for a comfortable place to camp, saw a group of friends, a family whom I have known all my life. They greeted us warmly and congratulated us on our engagement.

I relished this summer, our first house, our plans to get married in the fall. I had never been so happy, completely secure, and yet, in a peculiar way, acutely aware of life's fragility, as though intense happiness reminded me of our mortality. And I have always loved the sea, have always identified it with the happiest moments of my childhood summers on Cape Cod. Our friends' daughter reminded me of myself as a child. Her hair was bleached-out by the sun, her smooth backside was bare and tan, and she exuded freedom, running around the open beach, taunting the waves.

After twenty minutes in the sun we decided to go in for a swim. Both Jack and I have always loved to body-surf, but I had grown more cautious with age and had been frightened by a riptide the day before. But that was yesterday, and today the waves were big, there was no undertow, and the tide was low so that the water wasn't terribly deep. It is rare to be able to body-surf off Long Island, because the contour of the beach is irregular and precipitous. Generally the waves break much too close to shore to give you even a tiny ride.

Today was different. There is nothing more exhilarating than riding a wave, catching it at the perfect moment just before its swell turns into a cascading crest, fighting to stay out in front. I had always admired Jack's talent for catching the biggest or smallest wave, swimming with it and then riding it to the shore. I'm lazy and usually dive under as many as I ride in. I also chicken out. But today we were drunk with the ocean and sun. We stayed in the water until we were chilled, then baked on the beach and went back in the water again. By three thirty we decided to go home, to rest and shower before a Sunday-night cookout of steak and corn on the cob.

Jack decided to jog down the beach, and when I saw him in the distance ready to turn back, I ran to join him. We would take one last swim before leaving. The waves were getting bigger, and we both had one or two perfect rides. Then I dove under a breaking wave and, when I surfaced, turned to see where Jack was. I saw nothing but foam. Then his head popped up and he cried for help. I tried to run toward him and felt as though I were part of an anxiety dream where you try to run but cannot move your legs. But this wasn't a dream. The water fought my efforts to reach Jack quickly, and for a second I felt panic and heard myself cry his name.

It made no sense. It made no sense. It could have been me or either of our friends who had been swimming with us all day. Thank God for the people on the beach. I could never have pulled Jack out by myself. And the irony, I found out later, was that the curly-haired man did not know how to swim. And then there was Stanley, an elf of a man with sun-bleached hair and skin the color of molasses, who maternally brushed the sand away from Jack's eyes and kept telling him that everything was going to be all right.

Neither Jack nor I had ever looked better. We had spent a month's holiday in Mexico and California six weeks before, and the hot July sun had deepened our color. I remembered looking down at my body in the shade of the ambulance. My skin was smooth and brown, my breasts full, the bikini a little too small. Walking into the hospital, I felt naked and vulnerable. Everything was cool and clean inside, medicinal, sterile, but not unkind. I felt again I was part of a bizarre anxiety dream, the kind where you find yourself in a crowded restaurant having lunch with impressive-looking strangers and realize you are completely naked. I walked slowly next to Jack's stretcher, holding his hand. An X-ray technician, realizing I was uncomfortable, handed me a white coat. I watched them wheel Jack into the X-ray room and waited, no longer aware of how I looked or felt.

The X-ray showed nothing. Possibly, the doctors said, the vertebrae in the lower spine had dislocated and snapped back into place. Possibly. But Jack still couldn't move. I felt no relief. There is such a thing as contained panic, a condition akin to calm and born of ignorance, impotence, dread, and hope. Jack and I stared silently at each other as he was wheeled out of the X-ray department through the emergency lobby and into an empty, windowless room that looked like a cell.

I had to speak with the policeman who had accompanied us from the beach to the hospital. I saw the curly-haired man who had helped me pull Jack out of the ocean just an hour before walking toward me, our car keys and my red beach dress in his hands. I thanked him and asked if he would write his name down on a piece of paper.

The policeman rechecked the information I had given him on the beach. Yes, we were to be married in October and had rented a house for the season. I had debated for a split second on the beach telling the police that we were married because I was petrified that they might separate us. This same policeman, blond and baby-faced, was the first to diagnose Jack's "problem" as a broken neck, but I had still not made a connection between that and paralysis. The only person I remembered breaking his neck was Scarlett O'Hara's father in *Gone With the Wind,* and it had killed him. I was touched by the policeman's concern. He wished us luck, mentioned a case of a man whose house had fallen on top of him, had been paralyzed, and was walking a year later. . . .

They shaved Jack's head around his ears. He was describing what he could and couldn't feel to a nurse. I couldn't believe he was unable to move. He looked so healthy, his chest a dark rust color and his arms and shoulders muscular. On the beach when he told me he couldn't move his legs, I had refused to believe him and in a frantic gesture had tried to prop his legs up to prove he was wrong. The legs had collapsed.

They were going to put Jack into traction, and Dr. Spinzia explained that he would have to stay in the hospital for approximately six weeks. Six weeks! Jack was supposed to teach a night course at Columbia. What about his work . . . and I would have to arrange something with the office. I was still part of a scheduled existence where time is punctuated by plans, and fictitious futures are marked neatly into black books and calendars. I tried to call my father from the hospital, but he wasn't home. I left a message with his service: "Call immediately. There's been an accident."

A tall, horsy-looking blonde asked me to fill out an admission form for Jack. "I wonder how long Jack'll have to stay here," I said. "We're supposed to be married in October."

"Oh, don't worry," she said. "I bet you'll be a beautiful fall bride." She paused, but I didn't say anything. "Dr. Spinzia's a superb orthopedic surgeon, really outstanding." I didn't care. I wanted to go home and have the barbecue dinner we had planned.

My father called. I told him that we had been body-surfing, that Jack had been thrown by a wave and couldn't move, that the attending physician was a man named Joseph Spinzia.

"Are you all right?" my father said in his scratchy voice.

"I'm fine," I said. I felt better just hearing his voice. Ever since I was a little girl I always trusted my father, always went to him to discuss my problems. He was direct and honest but never cold. He was a doctor, but my father first. "Papa, don't worry about me. I'm really okay."

"Mama and I will drive out tonight," he said. "You stay at the hospital and figure we'll be there in around three hours."

"You don't have to drive out tonight. Really. I'll be fine."

They insisted on coming. I thought of going home alone to a dark, empty house. "Okay," I said. "I'll wait for you at the hospital."

A nurse warned me that Jack would be bleeding where the tongs were drilled into his head, but that everything was all right. Visiting hours were over, but no one said I had to leave. I walked to Jack's room and saw two nurses wheeling him toward me. For some strange reason the blood didn't disturb me. I only noticed how red and thick it was. Jack was asleep and I watched his belly heave up and down. The wounds in his head were still trickling in an irregular drip, like water from a broken faucet. He woke up for a moment but was too drugged to speak. I told him I would be close by. A nurse passed by me and said she hoped I didn't plan to spend the whole night at the hospital. No, I was just waiting for my parents to arrive. At that moment I saw my mother and father walking toward me. For the first time since the accident, I felt my throat constrict and my eyes fill up with tears. There was nothing to say. We just embraced.

I led Papa into Jack's room. Jack's eyes slowly opened and he smiled. My father put his hand gently on Jack's arm.

"Wow," he said softly, "you're really done up good. Are you in a lot of pain?"

Jack told him no and tried to explain what had happened. Papa told him not to speak, that he had looked up Dr. Spinzia before driving out and that he was a good man and also that the Southampton hospital was very good. His presence, his gaze, his tone were comforting. My mother came in for a short visit, and then my father said we should go, that Jack should get some sleep. I kissed Jack good-bye and he told me not to worry. I wanted to hold him. I kissed his mouth and nose and told him not to worry. I would see him in the morning. I left. As we walked down a long, quiet hall, my father put his arm around my waist and my mother held my hand.

It was 10:30 P.M. when we finally left the hospital. The house was black, and when I turned on the kitchen lights I saw the half-eaten English muffin, the remains of a late breakfast, and the cookies we had decided not to take to the beach. Something horrible had happened at four thirty that Sunday afternoon, but I didn't really know what. The house was exactly as we'd left it, and I felt strange being there without Jack. I walked into our bedroom, stared at Jack's shoes and slacks before picking them up off the floor. On the night table were his keys, wallet, and black notebook. Something horrible had happened at four thirty on July 12, and I was beginning to relate to it as one relates to a death.

I was glad my parents were with me, and yet their presence seemed strange. The little farmhouse in the middle of a green lawn in the middle of potato fields was Jack's and my first house together, and it embodied all my hopeless romanticism about being in love, getting married, and having babies. My father and mother in city clothes looked pale and tired. I realized that all I was wearing was my beach dress and that my tanned skin had a film of salt on it.

My father looked exhausted and said he was going to bed. He had to drive back to the city early that morning (it was almost one o'clock by now). He still had two babies to deliver before July 20, the date he and my mother were to leave for

Europe. For months they had been planning a trip to Brittany, down the west coast of France to Bordeaux. My younger sister, Annie, was already abroad and expected to meet them in Paris at the end of August. My mother and I went upstairs to make up the double bed in one of the extra rooms. When Jack and I had taken the house the previous March, we'd discussed how we would have friends out to share the weekends. It was a perfect house, simple, old-fashioned. It even smelled like the house I had lived in for fifteen summers on Cape Cod. "We can have the Wardenburgs out, and the baby can sleep in the room next to them. And the place is big enough so we won't get into each other's hair." Jack had laughed at my enthusiasm, my ability to rationalize anything I wanted badly enough. Yes, he loved the house, too, but he loved my childish joy about having it even more. It seemed ironic that now my mother and I were making hospital corners for a hideous emergency.

She wanted to sleep with me downstairs, but I wanted to be alone. I gave my father an alarm clock and kissed him good night. He didn't tell me not to worry. Mama and I went into the miniature green living room to talk. The room was so tiny, the furniture so small that anyone over five feet tall looked like a giant who had invaded a doll's house. I had stopped smoking a year before but found myself chain-smoking my mother's cigarettes. She told me I shouldn't start again. I told her that I didn't care. I suddenly realized I hadn't called Jack's parents in California.

I found Jack's black notebook and looked up their number. I stared at his handwriting. He had written all those notes, names, addresses, and phone numbers, and now he couldn't even move his fingers. I looked at the appointments he had scribbled down for the following week—a lunch date with Jon somebody that Monday, dinner with my Aunt

Mabel Tuesday night, a trip to Louisville the following Friday. I dialed his parents' number and his mother answered the phone. She was so happy to hear my voice that my immediate response was good-natured calm, as if I had forgotten why I was calling. "There's been an accident," I heard myself telling Libbie. "We were body-surfing this afternoon and Jack was thrown by a wave and hurt himself. . . ."

There was no hysteria or dramatic silence from her end of the phone. She wanted to know if he was in the hospital, whether he had broken anything. I told her that he was in traction, that the X-rays showed no fractures, that he wasn't in pain but that he couldn't move. I told her my parents were with me, that Papa had investigated the hospital and doctor, and I would call her the next morning to keep them posted.

The conversation was brief and, in an eerie way, detached. I hung up the phone and went back into the living room to rejoin my mother. The phone rang and it was Libbie again. Something had begun to sink in. After all, it was only ten o'clock in Los Angeles. Libbie and Lou had probably finished dinner and were sitting up reading when I called. I went over the details again, de-emphasizing the paralysis and re-emphasizing how good the care had been so far. The more rational I became in describing the accident, the more removed I felt from crisis. But as soon as I hung up the phone for the second time, I was swept up in a sea of exhausted nausea. I had to sleep.

When you have shared the same bed with someone for a long time, there is a special feeling of loneliness and dislocation when he is gone. I was scared to turn out the light, afraid of sleep and of waking up alone. I pulled the flower-print cover to the foot of the two single beds we had pushed together and adjusted the white ruffled curtains that had been twisted by the wind. I took off my red beach dress and stared at myself in the mirror. The light in our powder-blue bedroom was soft and yellow, and my skin and hair looked golden. The contrast between the suntanned and the white parts of my body accentuated my hips and made my breasts look round and firm. It was almost as if my own image comforted me, as if I were celebrating my own health and ability to move at will as much as I was indulging in vacant narcissism. Admiring my own body made me feel closer to Jack. There were many times when I realized he was lovingly watching me preen myself in front of the mirror, moments when I thought or pretended to think he was out of the room. And at those same times when he would tease me about my vanity, he would laughingly admit how fabulously sexy we both were. Perhaps part of the wonder at being in love is the total appreciation of oneself and unembarrassed confidence that because you are loved, you are beautiful.

I finally turned off the light, and as my eyes got used to the darkness I could see the silhouette of a fat elm tree standing defiantly alone in the middle of a flat field. I could smell the sea, I could even hear the waves breaking on the beach. The sea. It had always been a haven to me, a summer refuge. Now I hated it. I went over the events of our last swim in minute detail. In slow motion. Why did we go in? Why didn't Jack dive under the wave? Why did it happen and what was it? And then, my head pounding, I realized there were no whys.

I stretched my arms out to touch Jack's side of the bed. The sheets were cold on his side, but I could still smell his scent on the pillows. I thought of him in the hospital fastened by his head to a contraption that looked like a giant spit. I knew he was safe in the hospital, that I would see him the next morning, but that something had come abruptly to an end. I started talking to myself: "Everything's going to be all right; Jack, I love you. Please, God, let everything be all right."

As I said the words I started to cry. I tried to visualize his neck from inside, to *see* his spinal cord. Dr. Spinzia had said that if Jack's condition didn't change, he was going to call in a neurosurgeon. I wanted to *see* what had happened. I wanted to *see*. To understand.

jack

I awoke and a young black man in a white uniform was standing next to me. I asked him what time it was. He told me eight o'clock in the morning and that he had let me sleep an extra hour. I was still in my swimming trunks, still sandy. It flashed through my mind why the hell they hadn't taken my trunks off. At the time it didn't seem to matter. I was lonely and depressed and felt totally disoriented. It was Monday morning. I should be at work, but here I was in a hospital with no idea of how seriously I was hurt.

I couldn't turn my head sideways, and my neck was stretched so far back by the tongs and weights that I couldn't bend my head forward. I was staring straight up at the ceiling. The young man was leaning over me so that I could see him.

"What's your name?" I said.

"Clive. I'm a nurse's aide."

"Can I have something to drink? I'm thirsty as hell."

"I don't know," he said. "I'll ask. In the meantime this will help," and he rubbed my parched lips with a cotton swab that had been soaked in a sugary lemon substance. I licked my lips; it quenched my thirst a little but compounded the already awful morning taste I had in my mouth.

I told Clive, and he brought me some mouthwash in a cup with a straw. He tried to hand it to me. I instinctively reached for it but couldn't grip the cup. So he held it while I sipped, rinsed my mouth, and spit it into a metal tray, getting most of it on my chin. A nurse came in and said it was all right for me to have liquids, so Clive gave me a container of milk and a glass of orange juice. But he said he couldn't give me anything to eat. I didn't care because I wasn't hungry.

Another nurse came in and asked me to squeeze her hand. I held her hand but couldn't squeeze. She scratched the soles of my feet, just as the people on the beach had done, and I told her I could feel it. She said that was good. At the time, I was so high from the Demerol that it never occurred to me to ask why that was good. Did it mean the paralysis was not serious or that it was only temporary? I hadn't asked Joe many questions the day before, either. Somehow I knew he wouldn't commit himself to anything that early, so it would be useless to try to get into it.

I wished Mary were with me. I wanted someone to talk to. I was scared, lying there, waiting for doctors and nurses, all strangers, to get around to seeing me, waiting to find out what was wrong with me, waiting to find out what they were going to do with me.

I thought back to my first lonely days in the army. I remembered how I tried to keep busy while a lot of guys just lay on their bunks and stared up at the ceiling, waiting for whatever it was that was going to happen. Now, like them, I stared at the ceiling, scared, not fully comprehending what had happened to me, still replaying the wave in my mind, waiting for something to happen to me and wishing that someone would pay more attention to me.

The room I was in was very small. The walls were light green. The ceiling was made of large, white perforated plasterboard. My frame was next to the door and there was a large window on my right that faced the corridor. I could vaguely see the window but couldn't see out of it. My roommate, who was moaning softly to himself in his sleep like a hurt animal, was on my left. Next to him was a small window. I could see the light coming through but couldn't see out of it either. Not even the sky.

I thought it would be easier on Mary and her parents if they moved me into the city. And I'd be closer to work. I wondered if they could do that. The thought scared me a little because of all the horror stories I'd heard about the lack of care in New York hospitals. But then I realized that I had no idea whether the Southampton Hospital was any better or even if Joe was a good doctor. I dropped it. I was sure that Mary's father, Norman, was taking care of everything for me.

Joe came into the room. "How do you feel?" he said. "About as good as anyone can feel under the circumstances, I guess." It was true. I didn't hurt. I didn't feel sick. The tongs in my head didn't bother me, although they did feel a little strange. And I had no urge to go anywhere since I couldn't move. I was worried that they hadn't identified the trouble yet.

"What do you think is wrong with me?"

Joe pressed his hand on my belly. "Why you can't move? I don't know. But gas is accumulating in your belly. We're going to have to put a tube, a Levine Tube, down into you to suck it out."

A few minutes later a doctor, who, I thought, was Chinese or Filipino, came into the room.

"Relax," he said. "This might be a little uncomfortable, but it won't hurt."

He began pushing the tube into my nostril, but he hit a membrane and the tube got stuck. Then he tried the other side, but the tube got stuck again. He started to push harder. "That hurts!" I yelled. He didn't say anything. He just kept wiggling and pushing the tube. I started to panic. Then the tube somehow cleared the nasal passage.

"Swallow," he said, as he began shoving it down my throat and into my stomach. As soon as it was in, a brownish fluid began to flow out of me into a jar near my bed.

Then the doctor pulled out another tube and told the nurse to take down my swimming trunks.

"Relax," he said again. "This won't hurt."

"What are you doing?" I said.

"I'm going to insert this tube through your penis and into

your bladder so that it will automatically drain."

I had a flash. I remembered a boyhood friend, Bernie, telling me that the worst thing about his hernia operation was the pain when they shoved "this tube up my cock." I tensed as the doctor grabbed my penis and began inserting the tube. In a way I wanted it to hurt, I wanted to feel pain. But at the same time I was afraid.

I felt the tube go in, but there was no real pain. I could see the doctor's arms slowly pushing the tube farther and farther in. I waited for the pain. There was none. I felt the tube bend with my penis. I felt one final push and then the doctor looked as if he were tying the tube off, securing it to something.

I felt something, I thought. That's good.

Then a nurse brought in another bottle on a stand with a tube attached and inserted a needle into my arm—intravenous feeding.

The doctor and nurses disappeared. I tried to stay calm. The tube in my throat was a little uncomfortable, but it didn't really bother me, and I tried to concentrate on the brown liquid coming from my belly.

About mid-morning Clive and a couple of nurses came in. They took what looked like soft and furry sheepskins and covered me from my chin to my toes.

"What are you doing?" I said.

"We're going to turn you onto your stomach. If you're on your back too long, you'll get bed sores."

"What's such a deal about bed sores?"

"They're more than just sores. They're skin ulcers, which get infected and pussy."

Then Clive and one of the nurses picked up a large metal frame and placed it on top of me. My face was exposed except for my chin and forehead, which were supported by canvas straps. They strapped the top frame to the one I was lying on.

"Just like a ham sandwich," one nurse laughed. "Okay, now, we're going to turn you. Just relax and it won't hurt at all."

I didn't say anything. I felt strangely secure strapped in like that. Only the Levine Tube was a little uncomfortable. With Clive at my head and a nurse at my feet, they slowly began turning the entire frame like a spit. I tensed and my body slid a little sideways. My neck moved and I felt the bullets of pain shoot through my shoulders and into my arms. I screamed in pain, and they quickly finished the turn. When I was on my stomach, the pain stopped. I was staring down at the floor, my head supported by the two canvas straps, which were cutting into my chin and forehead.

"Get me out. Hurry," I pleaded.

They took the top frame and sheepskins off my back. That helped a little.

"How do you feel?" Clive asked.

"I slipped when you turned me. I think you hurt my neck." I could hardly talk. The straps kept cutting into my face and the Levine Tube was still very uncomfortable. I wanted to be turned back. "The straps hurt," I said.

Clive tried to adjust them for me, but it didn't help.

"Turn me back," I grunted. "I can't take any more."

"You've got to try it a little longer," the nurse said. "You've only been over five minutes and you must stay on this side for at least two hours."

Two hours. The pressure from the straps was killing me, and the Levine Tube was pressing against my larynx so that I could hardly talk. I tried to relax but couldn't. The sweat was pouring off me. A couple of the nurses walked out of the room.

"Don't leave. Turn me back."

"Five more minutes."

I tried to wait but couldn't. "Turn me," I screamed. I felt Clive putting the sheepskins on my back and strapping me into the frame. "Tighter," I ordered. Then they began turning me. I slipped again. The pain was excruciating. Finally I was on my back and the pain stopped. They unstrapped me and lifted off the frame and sheepskins. I lay there, staring at the ceiling, exhausted, gasping for breath. "The pain is incredible," I said to one nurse. "I slip around when you turn me. I want to see Joe."

"It's Dr. Spinzia's orders—every four hours."

"I don't care. I want to talk to him."

"He'll be by later." They all began to leave.

"Clive. How do I ring for help if I need it?"

He placed a buzzer in my hand and told me to push it. I couldn't. I couldn't squeeze that lousy little hospital buzzer.

"I can't," I said.

"Try," Clive said.

I tried. "I can't."

A nurse came in and told me that I was purposely put in this room because it was across from the nurses' station and that if I needed anything, I just had to yell. Then she left. The panic mounted. What if they didn't hear me? I waited about three minutes and yelled, "Nurse." With the tube in my throat, it was hard to yell. Nobody answered. "Nurse. Nurse." More time passed and then a nurse appeared.

"What do you want?" she said.

"What time is it?"

"About ten."

I waited for Mary.

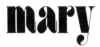

mary

It was just beginning to be dawn when my father woke me. He wanted me to lead him to the highway back to New York as he is notoriously bad at following directions in a car. I walked outside. The air was clean and cold and the sky a thin, ethereal blue. My feet were wet with dew and covered with freshly cut grass. My senses seemed anesthetized. I had an incredibly empty feeling, a hole in the pit of my stomach. The morning was beautiful but joyless. I was awake but still asleep, so out of touch with how I felt that I methodically and efficiently wiped the morning mist from the windshield, started the car, and led my father to the Montauk Highway. I was even careful to use my direction blinkers and keep an eye on Papa through the rear-view mirror. We waved good-bye to each other. Papa rolled down the car window and said he would try to drive out the following day. On the way back to the house I saw the sun rise over the flat horizon of potato fields.

When we had first started coming out for weekends in late May, the potato plants were tiny green specks. From the bathroom window I could see the perfectly straight rows rush toward the sand dunes like a series of railroad ties and converge at what looked like a single point in the distance. As the plants got fuller, the geometry of the landscape softened.

The kitchen was now filled with sunlight, and the early-morning chill had disappeared. I was so depressed that I felt queasy and resented the beautiful day.

I knew that I wouldn't be able to see Jack for hours and that it was still too early to call the city, so I tried unsuccessfully to fall asleep again. I thought about what I would say to Jack's boss and how I would manage to complete the files I was preparing for *Newsweek.* Just three days before, I had spent a hot, sticky day at Grossinger's interviewing some of the actors in *Taking Off* for a story on Czech film directors in

New York. That day was vivid in my mind but felt millions of miles away. My thoughts about "before the accident" might become an obsession. Just three days before, busily interviewing Buck Henry and Lynn Carlin, going home to fix dinner, making love, I had had no idea what was going to happen.

I heard my mother puttering around in the kitchen. She thought I was still asleep and was trying to make as little noise as possible. I joined her in the kitchen and she asked me how I had slept.

"Mary, you must eat something," she said. Her dark brown eyes reflected her concern, immediate and maternal—I had to have something in my stomach. I agreed but could only manage to swallow half an English muffin and some coffee.

I looked at the plastic clock over the icebox and realized that Jack's boss at NET was probably at work. Bill accepted the collect call without hesitation. It was unusual for me to call him, but his voice was friendly, almost welcoming.

"Jack's been in an accident," I said. "He's in the Southampton Hospital in traction. They don't know exactly what's wrong—we don't know how long he'll be away from the office."

As I was mouthing the words, I started to shiver, not from cold but from intense nervousness. I knew how excited Jack was about the new show that was to debut in January. He had spent one whole drive out to the country telling me about a concept he had for a new type of television format. It was important to him.

"Oh, my God," Bill said over and over. He kept telling me to tell Jack not to worry about work, that everything would be taken care of and that he would let the rest of the staff know what had happened.

"Please, tell Jack not to worry," he repeated. "And for
God's sake, if there's anything I can do, please call me. As
you know, we're in our house in Westhampton every weekend and . . . well, just anything we can do, just let us know."

As a child, I would occasionally imagine with terrible guilt
what I would do and whom I would turn to if my parents
died. Would I live with my Aunt Mabel or be adopted by my
parents' friends, the Ganzes, in which case I'd have an extra
three sisters and brother? Maybe I'd be like Sarah, the beautiful half-Indian orphan girl in *The Little Princess*, my favorite
childhood book. There was no doubt that I'd be excused
from school and that when I returned all the teachers would
be sympathetic and understanding. These hideous thoughts
always led to the same conclusion, in extreme cases to tears,
and most usually to the desperate hope that nothing would
happen, that as theatrical as these imaginings were, I loved
my parents and wanted to live with them forever, or at least
until I got married. Now my life, our life, was being threat-
ened by some inexplicable but very real catastrophe. The
childhood fantasy was now real life, a nightmare that I knew
I couldn't wake up from to find my life warm and safe again.
I knew exactly how I felt about my responsibilities to
work. I would let the office know what had happened, would
somehow finish my work on the story, but would stay near
Jack for as long as I had to. At that point, I truly believed
that there was a good chance that I'd be back in the city in
about ten days, working at the very least on a part-time basis.
As I heard the *Newsweek* operator answer the phone I began
to shiver again. I wanted to speak to my immediate boss, the
warm, pint-sized den mother of researchers whom I've
always had a special feeling for, but she wasn't there. So I
talked with another editor.

"This is Mary," I said. "I'm out on the Island and wanted to tell you that my fiancé has been badly hurt and is in the hospital."

Dead silence on the other end of the phone.

"I will finish my files today and give them to my mother. She can drop them off at the office early tomorrow . . . but I will not be in until we know more."

At this point he responded with a hollow, "Yes?" I could tell that he didn't believe me. He thought I was making up the story to get out of work, so I went into more detail, hoping he would believe me, but not really caring. I refused to play for sympathy, but I heard my voice crack and felt my eyes well up with tears.

"Listen, Jack can't move, and I don't think I will be back in New York for a week . . . I just don't know . . . maybe not for longer than that."

There was another silence but shorter and a little less suspicious than before.

"Well," he said matter-of-factly, "at least he's not a paraplegic, is he?"

"No, he's not a paraplegic. He's a quadriplegic."

Visiting hours didn't start until one o'clock, but by noon I couldn't wait to see Jack. I drove past the beach on the way to the hospital and recognized the spot where the ambulance had been waiting the day before. "This time yesterday . . ." I thought out loud. What was the point? Jack was waiting for me, and I felt an overpowering urgency to see him, to be with him.

I started to walk down the long green corridor that was now filled with sunlight and realized my legs were moving faster and faster, until I actually broke into a trot. I peered into Jack's room and hesitated a moment before going in. There was a tube in his nose. I remembered seeing my

1805921

mother right after a gall-bladder operation with that same tube in her nose. She was moaning, half-conscious and obviously in pain. I remembered having to leave the room because I felt faint.

Jack called my name. Somehow he knew I was there even though he couldn't see me. I bent over him and kissed his lips. His face was a mass of freckles. His wonderful blue eyes looked tired, and his healthy color seemed a fraud of nature. He had a sheet draped over him, and as I lifted it I thought it strange that he was still wearing his bathing trunks. I saw a plastic tube that ran from his penis to a plastic sack partially filled with urine. Nothing had bothered me before—not the blood, not the tongs in his head, not even the tube in his nose. But the sight of that plastic tube in his penis made my stomach sink. I asked Jack whether it had hurt when they put the tube in his nose.

"Yes," he said, "but it feels more uncomfortable now than it actually hurts."

I didn't want him to think I was upset, so I casually asked him whether the catheter hurt him. He said it didn't, and I pretended that I was glad. My mind started to race. It *should* have hurt him to have something stuck into his penis. A friend's father who had kidney stones had described the pain of having a catheter inserted into him as excruciating. Maybe I misunderstood him. Maybe it was the passing of the stones that was unbearable. But, no, I didn't think so.

I quickly told Jack that I had spoken to his boss, who had been wonderful. Jack's eyes looked straight ahead. He was thinking, not depressed, just thinking.

"Maybe they should get someone else," he said. "They need a healthy producer."

I told him to shut up, that he was being stupid. There was always that possibility, but now it was much too early to know and he shouldn't torture himself thinking about it.

Jack smiled at me and I bent down to kiss him. I didn't care about the roommate behind the curtain. Jack and I were so close, still so attracted to each other, still so sexually attuned. We loved. We made love with kisses. We spoke to each other in whispers, blocking out the sterile world that surrounded us. We looked so deeply into each other's eyes that we fused.

I spent a good part of the day making a list of things Jack wanted done—making calls, breaking dates, taking care of a world we were no longer a part of. I was tense with waiting. The doctors had taken new films of Jack's neck but still couldn't determine what was wrong. Not knowing made the wait more trying.

I had to call Jack's parents. My God, it was only four o'clock and I felt as if it should be getting dark already. I never felt panicked around Jack, but as soon as I entered that dirty, cream-colored phone booth, my heart started to beat at twice its normal rate. And then there was nowhere to sit, and I clutched the dimes, the yellow, now tattered piece of legal paper, my cigarettes, matches, and stub of a pencil, all the while trying to dial the operator. When she didn't answer, I'd wait patiently. My life was made up of waiting, and the fury I usually felt at the incompetence and stupidity of the Bell Telephone Company had disappeared. Or else was so buried by self-control that my heart was completely hardened to it all.

Finally I got through to Jack's parents, and his brother Dick answered. I was so happy to hear his voice. My instinct was to kid him as I had so often done before, but his voice was almost foreign to me, and the shock of hearing the sadness in his tone frightened me. I told him what was going on—nothing—but that the doctor seemed extremely capable. Dick hardly spoke. He seemed numb. I wanted to hang up the phone.

Night finally came, a clear, cold night for July. I walked into Jack's darkened room. He was asleep. I touched his arm, lightly ran my fingers across his chest.

"Hi, doll," he whispered. "How ya doin?"

"I love you, Jack. Everything is going to be all right."

He closed his eyes again and smiled. I didn't want to leave him but knew that he had to rest. Anyway, the loudspeaker in the hospital was already announcing the end of visiting hours. I kissed his cheek and told him that I would be back before I left the hospital. He heard me but kept his eyes closed. I knew he wasn't in pain and that he wasn't really sick, but his stillness spoke to me of danger. He was like an animal which has broken a limb and lies still, which instinctively knows that he must rest, that he cannot resist anyone's help because he is at the mercy of nature.

I heard my name being announced on the loudspeaker. Someone was calling me long distance. I didn't recognize the voice or the name on the other end of the phone, but whoever it was was nervous and excited.

"Look, Mary, I'm a friend of Jack's brother, Dick." The voice seemed disembodied, disconnected from a familiar face. "I'm a psychiatrist, and my brother-in-law is a neurosurgeon. I don't like what Dick tells me. It sounds like Jack's in bad shape and time is crucial now."

My head began to pound. Who was this person and why was he trying to shake me up? Why was he intruding?

"Listen, I know you're under a great strain, but why haven't they done a myelogram?" He stopped as though my silence indicated that he was upsetting me. "I wouldn't call if it weren't Jack's bod that is racked up."

I didn't know what a myelogram was, but the word bod really infuriated me. Jack's bod. What did he know about Jack's bod?

"My father has been checking up on everything that's

going on, and they are doing everything they can," I said curtly.

The voice interrupted me. "I understand," he said, "but it's a small hospital and . . ."

He was three thousand miles away, had no idea what was happening, and was trying to tell me that I should be scared. I was scared. I was petrified. I knew that he was calling because he was concerned and that his intentions were good, but his call seemed rude and pointless, almost a cry of fire in a crowded theater, and I resented him utterly and completely.

"There is nothing we can do now," I said, trying to gain control. "Jack can't be moved, and the neurosurgeon is coming tomorrow."

When I hung up the phone I was shaking. I looked up to see who had put his hand on my shoulder and saw my older brother, John. The sight of him, the surprise and emotional thanks that he was near me, made me want to cry. I knew he should have been in New York rehearsing a show. "Oh, John," I heard myself say, "it's all so awful."

I felt myself beginning to weaken, as much from exhaustion as from the lurking fear that Jack wasn't going to be all right. Mama lovingly put her blue cardigan around my shoulders as we drove toward East Hampton to find a place to eat. We drove in silence, and I thought how easily my mother would set the wrongs of my life right when I was a little girl. If something was bothering me, I would crawl into her lap and listen to her wise words and lullabies while we rhythmically swayed back and forth in her old mahogany rocking chair.

We stopped at a restaurant that had been decorated to look like a barn. The place was almost empty, and the candlelight and flowers on the tables reminded me of the depressing ambience of a dinner party where half the guests have forgotten to come. I still wasn't hungry, but Mama insisted I eat. John said he was starving and suggested I fill up my plate so he could eat what I didn't want. The sight of the food on my plate made the lump in my throat swell. I tried to swallow, but the lump wouldn't go down. The more I swallowed the greater the pressure became, like slowly rising mercury in a thermometer, until I could hold it in no longer. The relief of letting go was instantaneous. The tears rolled into my mouth as I talked.

"Oh, it isn't going to be all right," I sobbed. "I just have a terrible feeling that Jack's in danger. I just know it . . . I don't know. But I feel it."

The salty taste of my tears seemed to produce more tears. I tried to wipe my eyes with a napkin, and my brother and mother listened calmly. They seemed to know that silence was a greater solace for me than optimistic words.

"Why do you feel so sure?" my mother asked.

"I know . . ." I hesitated and tried to control my crying. "I know because of the catheter. I know because they don't catheterize a man unless it's serious." I hesitated again, frightened to admit what I knew was an even worse sign. "And Jack said it didn't hurt him when they put the tube in his penis."

My mother started to say that it didn't always hurt.

"Oh, yes. I know it should hurt," I interrupted. "I remember Tessa telling me how painful it was for her father when he had kidney stones. I know. I just know."

My mother said it didn't hurt her when she was catheterized for her gall-bladder operation.

"But you don't have a penis," John said.

We all laughed—even me, for a moment.

At one point during the meal I noticed a couple sitting at a table close to us. The woman was young and pretty. She had short blond hair and wore pearl earrings. She was about six months pregnant, and for a brief moment I hated her. I looked at her husband, who was wearing a madras jacket and rust-colored pants. They probably lived in Greenwich, Connecticut, and had dogs. I knew that they were aware that I was crying, but they never stared, and if they were uncomfortable, they never let on. I liked them for that. I had a flash of Jack and me making love . . . just two days before. We wanted to start to have a family soon, and I occasionally would ask Jack if we could try to get me pregnant the following May. When he said yes, I felt a rush of excitement and joy. Now, I thought, we might never be able to make love, much less have children, and I hated that couple for their seeming simplicity and happiness.

When we got home, I remembered that I had to type up some files for *Newsweek*. I was exhausted and couldn't have cared less about work, but I knew that I had promised, and that was that. John offered to type for me if I read the interviews aloud. I hoped they would take my mind off Jack, but they seemed so irrelevant. How differently I felt then, I thought to myself. How close I was to what was going to happen that weekend, yet how unsuspecting. It takes only a second to change or end a life. It takes longer than that to create one. The thought must pass through a billion mothers' and wives' minds when they hear that their husbands and sons have been killed in the war, but there the injustice is attributable to something, no matter how ugly, wasteful, or worthy the cause. I couldn't blame anyone for what happened, and it was still too early to feel cheated. Maybe I was lucky there was no one to blame, but I found myself cursing a God I hardly believed in.

I didn't cry myself to sleep that night, but I lay awake for hours. Something had come abruptly to an end. I knew that even then. There is a special conceit that lovers share, as though their happiness makes them superior to the rest of the world. And, in a way, this superiority is both real and illusory. We felt protected by our love, almost immune. Yet there was an early awareness that our love, like any love, was "two solitudes that bordered and saluted each other." I remembered a discussion we had had, lying peacefully in each other's arms. We were separate human beings, strong and vital, who had chosen each other because life was fuller that way. As Rilke had written, we were together to ripen, to become something in ourselves, to become world, to become world for our and the other's sake. And we knew that if something happened to one of us the other would go on. And then I remember we stopped and stared into each other's eyes. The thought of having to survive without the other was deeply disturbing but not frightening. We never said, "But nothing will happen," maybe we never even thought it. But we wished it.

When I awoke the next morning, I started to weep. Now I realized how alone I was; I was so frightened. No matter what my dreams had been the night before, sleep always came as a relief, a momentary escape from the harshness of the days, what I knew would stretch before Jack and me. When I'm happy, I welcome the days as though each morning were a microcosmic rebirth, a new chance . . . a new day. But when I opened my eyes that morning, my very soul seemed weighted in yesterday and the day before that, until my thoughts took me back to the ocean on July 12. "Oh, why did it have to happen?" I asked myself. The answer was always the same. "It happened because it happened."

I walked into the kitchen, and the sunlight hurt my eyes. Mama had left early in the morning, and I saw her empty coffee cup. I realized that I hadn't heard her leave. She had left me a note: "Darling, try to eat some breakfast. The car's at the station. See you tonight." I was glad she'd left the note, just as I was always glad when she left me notes when I was a little girl. Somehow her absence in those days had been more tolerable if I knew where she was. I remember that I used to call her name automatically when I walked into the house after school, and if she didn't answer I felt a rush of disappointment. I was glad she'd left me that note, and in an almost childlike way I looked forward to her coming home.

John came into the kitchen. He was wearing just his pants, and I noticed that his eyes and mouth were still a bit swollen from sleep. He saw that I had been crying, understood that I was still crying, though I was trying to hide it. He put his arm around my shoulders, and the gesture, so simple and wordless, seemed to say, "Cry, go ahead. It's good." I bent over the kitchen table, my hair covering my face. "I'll be all right," I kept repeating. "It's just so hard for me. . . . I'm always lousy in the morning."

As I started to walk down the long green hospital hall, I saw two nurses pushing Jack toward me. I grabbed his hand and kissed it. We were together again. It had been two nights that we'd slept apart, and though I had no choice but to accept the separation, I never really did accept it until I touched him. Ironically, I felt as though I were home again the second I was at his side.

jack

Mary was smiling when she came in and gave me a kiss. If the tubing bothered her, she didn't show it. I tried to tell her about their turning me that morning, but I could see she didn't understand. She said she'd called work for me and that Bill had been wonderful and had said not to worry about anything. I asked Mary to call my secretary and have her break or shift all my appointments to someone else. She left to make the call, and I thought about work.

The show wasn't due to go on the air until January. This was only July, but we'd already been working on it for six weeks. What should I do? I thought of a film producer I'd known in Canada who had broken his leg and had his staff assemble every day in his hospital room to screen and go over the film. I hardly felt like doing that even if it had been possible. Maybe they should get somebody else for the job. But I didn't know anything, Joe still hadn't found the cause of my paralysis, so I decided to wait.

That afternoon Joe came in. "I want to take another X-ray," he said. "There's an area of your neck we haven't been able to get a clear picture of. We'll do it in here so we won't have to move you."

A machine was wheeled into my room. Joe stood at my feet and grabbed my hands, which were lying by my sides.

"You're thick in the shoulders," he said. "I'm going to try to pull them down and out of the way, so we can get pictures of C-6, C-7, the two lowest cervical vertebrae. Ready?"

"Ready."

"Okay. Relax," he said and began pulling on my arms.

I tensed as he pulled. I felt those bullets shooting down my arms. I screamed. But Joe kept pulling while the X-ray was taken. Then he let go. He left with the technicians. A few minutes later he returned.

"We still can't get a clear picture," he said. "But as far as I can tell, nothing's broken."

Later that day Joe told me that if nothing changed by evening he was going to call a neurosurgeon in on my case.

"If you want to call your own doctor," Joe said almost apologetically, "I won't mind, but I have complete confidence in this man."

"What's his name?" I asked.

"Dr. Sengstaken . . . Dr. Robert Sengstaken."

I told Joe about the pain in my neck and arms when they turned me. He said it might be painful, but that it wasn't doing any damage and that I had to get off my back and onto my stomach every four hours.

"But I know the turning is doing further damage to my spine," I said.

"As long as you're in traction, Jack, it's impossible for the turning to hurt you. . . . If it's so bad, I'll hold off on the turning until we find out exactly what's wrong."

That night the older man in the bed next to mine was alternately moaning and delirious. I couldn't see him because the curtain around his bed was drawn, but when the nurses tried to roll him onto his side to bathe him he screamed in pain, swearing at them, begging them to stop, yelling that he couldn't stand it. I wanted to yell at them to stop, too, but I didn't. They got him over on his side and bathed him. Then they rolled him back while he begged them to go slowly. When the nurses left, I tried to talk with him, but it was impossible. When the night nurse, Swanee, came in, I asked her who he was.

"You're in with a celebrity," she said. "He's been written up in all the newspapers. He's a famous jewel thief—eighty years old. Tried one job too many, chief. Got caught out here in one of these swank houses, panicked, fell down a flight of stairs, and broke his hip."

Toward morning he woke up. "Where am I?" he said.

"You're in the Southampton Hospital," I answered.
"What am I doing here?"
"You're pretty badly hurt. I think you've got a broken hip.
You fell down some stairs, and they brought you here.
You've been delirious for the day and a half I've been here."
"I shouldn't be here at all," he said. "I was in a hospital in
Baltimore. I've been kidnapped. Call the FBI. Please call the
FBI."
"The FBI?"
"They're as powerful as the NKVD," he said.
"Listen, I can't move," I said. "But I'll call the nurse and
tell her to call the FBI."
"Don't do that," he said. "It was the nurses who kidnapped
me."
I wanted to laugh but couldn't. He was delirious. I was
paralyzed. But I thought if I could keep him talking, maybe
he'd tell me where he'd hidden his money. "Listen," I said,
only half kidding. "I can't call the FBI. But maybe if we pay
the nurses off, they'll call them. But I don't have any
money."
"I don't either," he said. "Call the FBI."
"You must," I said. "You've made all this money."
"I don't have any money. Call the FBI," he insisted.
I felt like a cop grilling a burglary suspect. I kept at it for
another few minutes, but he stuck to his story and kept asking me to call the FBI. It was ludicrous. I couldn't believe
what I was doing, so I finally gave up and tried to change
the subject. But he only babbled on about being kidnapped,
so I just shut up and tried to sleep.
Joe looked different when he came in to see me the next
day. The uncertainty was gone. He'd made up his mind
about something.
"I've talked to Dr. Sengstaken," he said. "He's coming out

here tonight. We're going to try to get a better X-ray, and if we can't, we'll take a myelogram. We inject a fluid into the spine and then trace it."

Neither Mary nor I said anything, and I think our silence made Joe defensive. He repeated that he didn't want us to think he was stubborn or inflexible and that we could still call in our own doctor if we wanted to. After Joe left, Mary said she had already spoken to her father and that he had heard of Sengstaken and thought he was excellent.

Sengstaken was supposed to arrive at four o'clock. Mary read to me and we talked. I tried to be cool. I didn't want to scare her or me. But as the afternoon wore on, I got more and more nervous. I wasn't scared that they might have to perform an operation or conduct a myelogram. I wasn't even scared of being X-rayed again. I just wanted to get on with it, whatever "it" was. At five o'clock Sengstaken still hadn't arrived. Mary said she wished he would hurry. We were both tense as we waited for him.

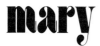

mary

We continued to wait anxiously, knowing that the longer the mystery lingered in everyone's mind, the more painful the waiting was—maybe even dangerous. At about eleven thirty we had been told that Sengstaken would be arriving at four o'clock. Apparently, he traveled around Long Island in a helicopter and had a short-wave radio in his car. I was relieved that he was finally coming, and when he still hadn't arrived by five, I found myself praying that he'd come soon. I was afraid Jack would see that I was nervous, even though I was controlled and calm on the surface.

"Don't worry, baby," he said softly. "He'll be here. Are you tired? Maybe you should go home and rest."

I told Jack I was fine and wanted to wait. Sengstaken would be here any minute. I could tell that Jack was anxious for him to arrive, anxious for him to get on with it. I could also see that he was frightened.

John arrived at around five and was talking with Jack when I thought I saw a man who must be Sengstaken. I remember that he looked tremendous to me, maybe six feet three inches tall, and handsome in a roughhewn way. When I saw him go into the nurses' station and look at what I thought was Jack's chart, I was sure it was he. I wanted to introduce myself. I wanted him to know who I was—Jack's girl and a doctor's daughter. I wanted him to be nice, but he seemed different from anyone, any doctor, I'd ever met. He was wearing an ugly summer suit, the type that shines too much, a yellow-brown fabric that borders on being cheap even though it isn't. He was wearing an almost aqua-colored shirt that I thought particularly unattractive. The clothes looked as if they belonged to another man, maybe a salesman. But I watched Sengstaken move, and even from a distance he commanded respect. He hardly spoke and seemed to move with incredible swiftness, but never seemed harried or rushed. When I saw he was alone, I walked over to him.

"Dr. Sengstaken," I said meekly. "I'm Mary Pleshette, Jack's fiancée."

He shook my hand, and I remember that I felt dwarfed by him as his huge hand enveloped mine. He didn't say anything. He didn't smile. I felt the same kind of fear I'd experienced on the beach—I might be separated from Jack. I might be pushed out.

"Excuse me," he said and shifted his attention to Jack's chart. I watched him scan the information as if he already knew what had to be done. He never sat down, never wasted a move. Everything about him seemed to say, "Let's get going."

There was no more waiting now. Things happened so quickly that we hardly knew what was going on. I felt at times that my presence was being tolerated by the doctors, that they would have preferred my not being so close. But they seemed to understand that I needed to be there and that Jack wanted me close by. If I felt Sengstaken was ignoring me, I didn't mind. Just as long as he didn't ask me to wait outside.

Joe arrived from nowhere. I saw him by Sengstaken's side. He was nervous and uncomfortable, as though Sengstaken's authority disturbed him. I wasn't allowed inside the X-ray room, but I tried to stand close by so I could hear what was happening. Sengstaken's voice was serious but kind. I thought I heard him tell Jack to relax. When he walked from the X-ray room to a small office nearby, I tried to accompany him from a distance. I dreaded their telling me to go away. They never did. I felt rigid, so desperate to find out what was wrong that my neck and eyes hurt from strained concentration.

I never took my eyes from Sengstaken. They had taken two films and still couldn't get a good picture of Jack's neck. Sengstaken was annoyed with the X-ray technician.

"You'll have to do better than this," he said.

Then they smiled when they clipped the third X-ray up against a lighted milky glass frame.

"We really got it," one doctor said.

"We sure did," Joe responded, and he seemed delighted too.

I thought everything was fine. They couldn't be so happy if it was bad. But I didn't really know, and I turned to John in the hope that he would understand what everything meant. He just raised his eyebrows quizzically. No one said anything. No one came over to me and said, "Everything's fine," and I thought I would burst with tension.

Sengstaken turned to me and said, "Would you mind coming in here?"

I followed him into a small blue conference room and watched him clip the X-ray of Jack's skull and neck onto a long lighted board. It was a side view. John was standing next to me.

"What is it?" I blurted out. I was frightened again. I waited for Sengstaken to speak, and I stared at the picture of an unfamiliar, surrealist skeleton that was Jack.

"It looks very bad," Sengstaken said. "He's broken and dislocated his sixth and seventh vertebrae."

He pointed with the eraser tip of a pencil. He helped me count as he moved the pencil downward.

"One, two, three, four, five . . . you see . . . they're all in place."

He didn't have to help me any more. Six and seven were at least a half-inch out of place, shoved forward toward Jack's jaw. There was a brief silence, and I could feel everyone's eyes glued to me, waiting for me to say something. I was sitting now, and I was numb. I felt suspended, almost weightless, as though I were floating in an alien world.

"Will Jack be able to walk again?"

Sengstaken was sitting on a desk top with his feet on a chair. His eyes were cold.

"No. He will probably never walk again."

The words seemed to echo in my head. I felt lost, completely alone. I felt as if I were drowning, or maybe I had already died. I saw my own eyes staring at me—vacant, pleading eyes.

"Why? Why are you so sure?"

Sengstaken came over and sat down next to me. He pointed to the X-ray and said in a soft, calm voice, "The spinal cord runs through the vertebrae. When Jack hit his head, those two vertebrae were pushed forward against the cord and hooked on to each other. The cord was probably severed or, if not, irreparably bruised and torn." He waited for me to say something. But I didn't. "You see, the spinal cord is like a telephone cable, and like the individual lines that run through it, the nerves carry messages from the brain to the muscles." Again he paused for a moment and then went on. "But unlike a telephone cable, once the spinal cord is torn, it can't be mended. . . . The result is permanent paralysis."

It was irreversible. Jack was paralyzed from the neck down. I quietly, almost politely, asked Sengstaken to stop. "Please. Just let me cry."

I buried my head in my arms and for the first time in three days wept without any desire to hold back. I felt my shoulders sag, my breast heave, and I held on to Sengstaken's left hand that was resting on the table in front of me. I pressed it to my forehead and felt myself gripping onto it. No one spoke, and Sengstaken made no effort to draw away from me. I felt him hold the back of my head in his right hand, and at one point he smoothed my hair. I told him I'd be all right. John, who sat next to me, kept mumbling, "Horrible. It's so horrible," while he gently rubbed my shoulder.

"Is there any chance he will recover?" I asked meekly. Sengstaken shrugged and said, "I seriously doubt it . . . but there are always miracles."

Nobody said anything for a few moments. Then Joe said, "I don't agree with Sengstaken." I was surprised that Joe would say this with both Sengstaken and me in the room. I looked up and saw that Joe meant what he was saying, that he wasn't trying to ease my sorrow. "I can't tell you why I feel this way, but I do. I don't think the cord has been severed."

"What are you going to tell Jack?" I asked.

Sengstaken said they wouldn't tell him anything, not unless he asked.

"How can you lie to him?" I asked.

"We won't lie to him. We will tell him everything he wants to know when he asks."

The "he" was separated from Jack. The "he" was someone I didn't know.

"You can't tell a man unless he asks that he will never walk again, that he will be paralyzed for the rest of his life at this point," Sengstaken continued. "If you did that, you would destroy any hope. And that's the only weapon now."

Sengstaken paused and looked sternly at me.

"He can't see you cry, Mary. He can't see that you are upset."

Sengstaken explained that they would try to unhook the vertebrae with traction, that they would add up to sixty pounds of weight to avoid having to operate. I waited while he disappeared into the X-ray room. He came back with another X-ray and quickly stuck it up on the lighted glass. Sengstaken and Joe studied the picture in absolute silence.

"We need another ten pounds," Sengstaken said. He went back into the X-ray room. Another ten minutes passed. He came back with another X-ray. "One of the vertebrae snapped back," he said. He had marked every X-ray with a red wax pencil in the order it had been taken, and I could see the difference in the latest picture. Mindlessly, I stared at the X-ray. I could *see* inside Jack's neck, but it was someone else to me. I felt as if I were in the midst of the movie Z. I remembered the scene where the lawyer sees the X-rays of Lambrakis, and I felt the pounding of that unrelenting music in my head. I was part of a movie. I was trying to un-ravel some weird, suspenseful mystery. The only difference was that my "husband" was not dead.

"Let's add some more weight," Sengstaken said. "Maybe we can get the second one back in place." He went into the X-ray room. It seemed like an endless, monotonous parade.

I was aware that someone had walked into the room. I turned and saw my father and mother. They didn't know anything, but they knew everything. I felt like crying again but couldn't. Sengstaken and Joe came back into the room. Sengstaken shook my father's hand and stuck a new X-ray up against the light. I half listened to the conversation be-tween Joe and Sengstaken, but nothing seemed to register any more. I dimly heard Joe say, "If we do that, we'll have to wire the sixth and fifth, and that won't work. What do you think?" It all sounded like a foreign language to me, but I was beginning to understand that the second vertebra hadn't snapped back, that whatever they were doing wasn't work-ing. Sengstaken didn't answer immediately. Finally he broke the silence and slowly turned to us all.

"We'd better get going. We have to operate."

I was standing in the pink-tiled ladies' room staring at my face in the mirror. I was still suntanned, and my hair was stiff with the salt water I still hadn't washed out for three days. My mind was the color of a hazy white day just before

it snows. I splashed some water on my face, and it felt hard
and cold. My eyes were swollen, and the water seemed to
soothe their burning. I looked again at my face. It *was* me,
not somebody else.

As I approached the X-ray room, I saw Sengstaken talking
with my father. I went up to them and said I was all right,
that I wanted to see Jack. Sengstaken led me into the room.
Jack's shoulder muscles were bulging from the stress of all
those weights. He looked like a healthy animal trapped and
tied down before being shipped off to a zoo.

"They're going to have to operate, baby," Jack said.

He asked Sengstaken to explain to me what was happening. He really didn't know what I knew, and I no longer
wanted to tell him.

Everyone seemed to be scurrying around. Joe and Sengstaken had disappeared to get something to eat before the
operation, and Jack was wheeled back to his room. A nurse
came in and gave him an injection. "This will relax you," she
said. "And it'll make your mouth real dry." The hospital
seemed deserted, the visitors were gone, the hall lights had
been dimmed, and the place stank of silence. When I looked
into Jack's eyes, I wasn't frightened. He asked me to get my
father.

"Do you think I have to be operated on?" Jack asked
calmly. "Do you think they're doing the right thing?"

"They know what they're doing," Papa said. "They have to
clean you up and straighten out those vertebrae. They have
to get the pressure off the cord." He paused. "Nobody goes
into the neck unless they have to. And I have confidence in
Sengstaken, and Spinzia's an excellent man."

Papa asked Jack if he wanted him to call his parents. "I
think we should," I remember Papa saying. Jack seemed
frightened for a minute, as though the realization of his
parents' coming meant that the operation was dangerous,

but no one said anything. "I guess you'd better," Jack said after a pause, and the fear lingered in his eyes.

A nurse came into the room with another injection. They were ready to wheel him into the operating room. I knew the nurses wanted me to leave, but I wouldn't go. I felt riveted to Jack's side. I wanted them to go away. I wanted more time, but they started to push the hard, narrow rack out of the room. I walked next to Jack, and a second before they pushed him behind two heavy swinging doors, I asked the nurses to stop. "Please, just let me kiss him good-bye," I said and didn't really understand the "good-bye." I told Jack I would see him when he woke up from the operation. I told him I loved him. I told him everything was going to be all right. I watched them push him into a large, cellarlike room, and I saw a group of people dressed in green wheel him out of sight. I felt an empty hole where my stomach was, and the forbidding doors closed.

My father put his arm around my shoulders as we walked out the automatic emergency doors of the hospital. I started to cry without knowing it. "Could Jack die?" I asked.

I felt my father's hand tighten around my arm. "Yes."

We waited in the green silence of that tiny farmhouse living room. My father looked at me solemnly. "You mustn't feel guilty if there's a part of you that wants Jack to die," he said. "Jack's an active, alive man, and if he's completely paralyzed for the rest of his life, that could be worse than dying."

I nodded but didn't say anything. I thought of life without Jack, and my stomach twisted itself into a knot. I pictured myself alone and saw myself, a specter of a person, closing the door to our apartment, putting Jack's suits and ties into huge suitcases. I thought of going home again, of sleeping in my single four-poster bed, waking up to a past that I was no longer a part of. I thought of life without Jack, having to meet new men, having to be on the make again, and the

/

thoughts exhausted me. The faces of old boyfriends floated in front of me like helium balloons. And then, quite methodically, I thought of all the men I had ever fantasized about who would be available to me.

I felt myself sinking into my past, a past that had never been so happy until I'd met Jack. And then I remembered that someone once told me that if you stretched out on your back in quicksand and tried to float, you wouldn't drown. "I don't want Jack to die," I said to myself. "I want more than life for Jack to live." As I uttered the words, I felt immediate relief, and with relief I felt hope, and with hope a surge of strength.

jack

I dreamed I was calling for Mary. Then I realized I was awake and Mary was next to me. She bent down and kissed me.

I don't remember feeling pain, but Mary says that the first thing I said was how much I hurt. Then I asked her what time it was, and she told me it was after midnight.

"And the operation?"

"It went well. Everything's okay," she said.

"Where's Joe?" I asked.

"He went home."

I was hurt. I didn't understand why he wasn't there. Didn't he care? I had a lot of questions to ask him. A nurse came over to us, and Mary said she had to go. She kissed me good-bye, and I fell back into a drugged sleep.

I was awakened by two nurses. It was still night, and they were covering me with sheepskins, furry sides down, from my shoulders to my feet. Then they placed the metal frame over me. They strapped it down so that I was sandwiched between the sheepskins and frames. I began to get frightened. They were going to turn me onto my stomach.

"Joe said I wasn't to be turned," I said.

"It's doctor's orders, Mr. Willis."

"But I've just been operated on."

"This won't hurt you."

"Call Joe. Please. Just call Joe."

"It's doctor's orders," they said, "four hours on your back, Mr. Willis, two hours on your stomach."

Two hours! I hadn't lasted ten minutes the first time. I gritted my teeth and waited for the pain as they turned me, but there was none this time, and I realized the operation must have relieved the pressure on my spinal cord.

I lay there in the dark, staring down into blackness. The straps cut into my forehead. I tried to sleep. I couldn't. I tried thinking about work, but I couldn't concentrate. All I could feel was the straps. I heard the nurses quietly move around the darkened room. I cried out. There was no answer.

"I can hear you," I yelled. "I know you're there."

No answer.

"Turn me back. My head is killing me."

"You've only been over five minutes, Mr. Willis," one of the nurses said, and the other one came over and rubbed my back and said I had to try to take more.

For the first time I felt the total impotence of my position. I understood for the first time what it really meant to be paralyzed. My frustration gave way to rage. "Goddamn, son-of-a-bitch. Turn me. I can't stand it," I screamed.

From the darkness came the answer: "We can't. Doctor's orders. Two hours on your stomach. You've only been over ten minutes."

Orders. It was like the goddamn army. Would those automatons let me suffer for two hours? I tried to wait but finally screamed again. "Get the doctor. Call Joe. It's crazy. I hurt. I can't stand it."

And then, miraculously, the nurse who had rubbed my back came out of the darkness and began placing the sheepskins on my back. I could hardly stand it. "Hurry," I said. She put the frame over my back, strapped me in, and without saying a word, rolled me over onto my back. "Get the frame off me fast."

She did and I relaxed and fell asleep. I dreamed I was running full speed down a hill. About halfway down, a fist materialized and smacked me full force right in the face. When I was a kid playing football in the street, I'd gone out for a pass and run into a lamppost and had been knocked cold. That's what the sensation was in the dream. I took a few more steps, and it hit me again and again and again.

I woke up dripping wet from my own sweat. I waited a

few minutes until I calmed down and then went back to sleep. The same dream began again. I was running downhill and got hit in the face over and over again. That dream is clearer to me today and more frightening than the accident itself.

I couldn't get back to sleep. I tried to piece together the events just before they operated on me. Sengstaken had told me then that two vertebrae in my neck, the lower two, were fractured and dislocated, the same two Joe had tried to get a picture of in my room the day before. They had been pushed forward and had locked together, causing pressure on the spinal cord, which accounted for the paralysis. To snap them back into place and relieve the pressure on the cord, they first had to be unhooked.

"We don't want to operate," Sengstaken said. "We'll have to roll you over for the operation, which could be dangerous."

I thought about being turned in my bed the day before and the pain in my arms. I wondered if any damage had been done then. I knew it was the wrong time to ask and that they wouldn't tell me even if they knew.

"We're going to add more weight to your head," Sengstaken said. "We're hoping to stretch you out and pull the vertebrae free of each other." He walked behind me and added weights to the twenty pounds already suspended from my head. "That's ten more pounds," he said. I lay there waiting, not knowing what to expect. I felt the added weight pulling on my body but felt no pain. Then I heard a snap and said, "I think it's back in place." They took another X-ray and disappeared into another room. I waited, thirty pounds of dead weight stretching my dead body. They came back in. "Only one vertebra's snapped back," Sengstaken said. The other one was still locked. "Let's try another ten pounds."

He added the weight, and we waited, expecting another

snap. After ten minutes, when nothing had happened, they took another X-ray and disappeared again. I made small talk with the X-ray technician, and Mary's father and brother came into the room.

"Where's Mary?" I asked.

"She's outside."

Sengstaken came back in. He stepped behind me, and I thought he was going to add more weight. Instead, he told me to relax and put his huge hands under my shoulders and tried to stretch me out farther by lifting and pulling my head toward him. I could feel the desperation in the effort and knew we had reached the end of the line. I let him try a couple of times, and finally I said, "I guess we've had it."

"I guess so," he said. "I think we have to operate."

"Let's get on with it," I said. But first I wanted Mary to know what was happening. I made him bring her in to explain everything that had happened and what was wrong with me and why they had to operate. I wanted them to know how close Mary and I were and that it was important to both of us that we go through this together. What I didn't say was that I needed her, that she had to know what was happening because at some point we were still going to have to make a decision about whether or not we were going to be married.

Joe brought her in. We smiled at each other, and then I said, "Hon, they're going to have to operate. You tell her, Doctor."

I listened while he explained what had happened to my vertebrae and spinal cord and why they had to operate. Her expression didn't change, she just kept nodding as if she understood, and she didn't ask any questions. Then she held my hand. I felt very close to her, and I was proud of the way she was handling everything. So was Joe, I guessed, because he suddenly said, "You kids are very brave. Don't think we haven't noticed. You're going to need to be even braver in the next few days."

The sun was finally up, and now I found myself objectifying all that was happening to me, the same as I had on the beach. I was looking down at myself, not quite believing it was happening to me. The day before, I had been happy to see Sengstaken. It meant that two days of waiting and wondering were over. I was even relieved when they finally got the X-rays and found the fractures. At least we knew what was wrong. And as crazy as it seems, I was relieved that they were operating. At least we were doing something.

But now it was the morning after the operation and I still couldn't move. The night before, Sengstaken had told me that all the damage was done to my spinal cord the second I hit my head on the sand. If my cord had been severed, the operation could relieve the pressure but could not bring back my movement.

I waited for Joe and tried to frame the questions I would ask him, like what did they find when they opened me up. But when Joe came in, I just blurted out, "Will I walk again?"

"Sengstaken doesn't think so," he said.

The blood rushed out of my head and I felt my heart sink.

"What are the odds?" I asked.

"About ten per cent," he said.

"And you. What do you think?"

"I don't know," Joe said. "I'm more optimistic."

I didn't really hear him. I rushed on. "Can I fuck?"

"Probably. But you wouldn't feel anything."

"Can I have kids?"

"I don't know. An erection doesn't mean ejaculation." Joe smiled. "Those were the same questions Mary asked."

Mary. So she already knew. I was glad because I didn't

want to have to tell her. The night before, when Joe had awkwardly attempted to help us by telling us how much everyone admired the way we were acting and how we were going to need all our courage in the days ahead, it had cheered me a little to get his recognition, but now it didn't seem to help. Now I searched for answers. But what? I sank lower and lower. I couldn't speak.

Joe began talking quietly. "The odds are against you," he said. "But there's some room for hope. When we opened you up, we could see that the cord was intact."

I pressed him. "Well, then what's wrong?"

"Sengstaken's pessimistic because of the paralysis and because he ran his finger down the cord and felt an indentation. He thinks that means a whole group of nerves within the cord have been severed . . . but I don't know. It could just be a temporary indentation, like the kind you get when you sit for a long time in a chair with slats."

"When will we know who's right?" I said. "When will movement begin to return if it returns at all?"

"In around two to three weeks," Joe said. "Not before then." He paused. "Even Sengstaken doesn't know for sure if the cord was severed. If it's only badly bruised, you should begin to get return when the swelling goes down. Give yourself a chance. If you still can't move after three weeks, then . . ."

Then? What then? What was I going to do? How was I going to deal with it? I couldn't even commit suicide. I couldn't move. Would Mary help me? Would Joe help me? It was all too dumb, all beyond comprehension.

I looked at him. He stared back. I was sure he was reading my mind. "I've got to see another patient," he said. "I'll see you later."

mary

When I opened my front door on a Tuesday evening in March, I thought Jack looked older than I had imagined he would be. But I was immediately comfortable with him and almost inadvertently took his arm as we waited for a taxi. When I realized that my hand was neatly resting on his, I made a conscious effort to keep it there. I was testing myself, testing Jack. I was saying, "This is the way I am, and I'm sick to death of first-date protocol."

I wore a light blue sleeveless dress and the beige Gucci shoes I'd bought the previous summer—the shoes which I'd saved twelve dollars on by buying them in Italy but which now killed my feet. I had suspected from his phone voice that Jack wasn't from New York, and I was now sure that my suspicions were right, from the thin black tie and cloddy shoes he wore. I was disturbed that I even noticed, much less cared about his clothes, but he was unlike anyone I had ever dated. I was the one who always had a fantasy that the man I'd marry would speak fluent French and that we'd have lots of beautiful, bilingual children. Jack didn't fit that mold.

We had dinner in the Village and I talked about how bored I was at *Newsweek,* how I longed for a job that would utilize all my energies. Jack listened. He often leaned forward on his elbows to hear me better. He seemed interested. I talked about the newness of being on my own, the incredible difficulty of learning to be alone. I talked about my family and he spoke about his. California seemed very far away. I had never been to California. After dinner we walked around the Village and Jack casually put his arm around me. We took a cab uptown and stopped at a bar near my apartment. Jack described his experiences, making films in the South, and I asked him whether he had been afraid. "No," he said. "I was much more frightened in Appalachia." Mississippi, Kentucky . . . AMERICA. He didn't fit the ideal image, but I liked him. I really liked him.

At one point I adjusted the barrette in my hair, and Jack asked me to leave my hair down. We walked back to my apartment and climbed up the four flights of stairs. Before I had time to worry about the usual first-date-good-night awkwardness, he grabbed me and kissed me hard on the mouth. I remember that I felt like a comic strip character with a big "WOW!" hovering over my head. When I closed the door, I was smiling.

I was smiling now. We were different people then, but those two strangers were a part of us. I lay quietly waiting to be called to go back to the hospital. By midnight I still hadn't received word but could wait no more.

Jack was in the Intensive Care unit, a large room with only a few beds. It was so quiet that even the sound of a footstep seemed an intrusion. A nurse in a green uniform led me to where Jack was sleeping. But he wasn't really sleeping, just resting. He looked as though he had been beaten; his cheeks were swollen, his eyes puffy and bruised. He could hardly speak, and I tried to quiet him as he struggled to talk to me.

"I hurt. Oh, Mary, I hurt so much," is all he said.

I hesitated before kissing him, afraid of hurting him more. The tube in his nose sucked a brown liquid and spit it into a bottle attached to his bed.

"You're okay, Jack. Don't talk. Everything is going to be all right. I love you. Just try to sleep."

Jack wanted to know what time it was. I told him midnight. He asked to see Joe. I told him that he'd gone home. I wanted to hold Jack's hand, to sit quietly by him and stay the rest of the night. A nurse came over to me and said I had to leave.

Jack was alive. The panic and fear had vanished. In its place was a calm, so real and solid that I understood I had passed through the nightmare and was now so firmly rooted in the present that nothing seemed to scare me. I knew nothing except that Jack was alive, and that knowledge seemed to steer me like an invisible rudder.

I drove slowly back to the house. The air was misty, and everything was quiet, still, soft. I could see the farmhouse from the road. My mother had left the kitchen light on. I parked the car and stared at the house. I was going home to my parents, and I felt a little like Emily in *Our Town*, traveling backward in time to her thirteenth birthday.

I had moved in with Jack about six months after I met him. I kept my little apartment but never went there except to mess it up the day before the cleaning lady was due to clean. Jack never spoke to me about marriage, which bothered me only when my mother asked me what our plans were, or told me that by all means I should not give up my apartment. I remembered telling her not to worry. I was living with Jack because *I* wanted to, and I wasn't concerned about getting married, so why was she? All these worries seemed laughable now.

I thought about how happy everyone was the night we announced we were getting married. It was my twenty-fourth birthday, a ridiculously special day for me every year, with a family celebration that always included gifts, poems, and my favorite dinner of roast beef and a strawberry shortcake for dessert. But this birthday was golden. Jack and I had decided to surprise everybody with the news.

Jack raised his glass of champagne. "A week ago today on Fisherman's Wharf in San Francisco, over a plate of cracked crab, I asked Mary to be my wife. . . . And she said yes." No one knew whether to drink the champagne or kiss us. There was a happy commotion—my wonderful Aunt Mabel, who had once broken all the windows in her courtyard trying to kill some noisy pigeons with a slingshot, cried, my brother kissed Jack, my mother kept repeating, "Oh, how marvelous, oh . . ." and my father glowed. And once the gleeful surprise had passed, I was bombarded with questions of when and where and by whom.

I realized a few weeks later that the knowledge that Jack and I would actually be husband and wife was giving me a phantom security, but I didn't want to wait five months. I wanted to be married right away. At times I felt a strange urgency, as though I were scared that waiting was an invitation to some unknown interference. I told Jack that I wished October weren't so many months away. But it was ironic, as I was the one who, for some reason, had always wanted to be married in the fall. Jack laughed and rocked me in his arms. We were sitting on the soft, smooth lawn in back of the house, facing the open, rambling potato fields. We waited for the sun to disappear and watched the colors of the country gently fade into the cool grays of dusk. For a moment I realized how very small we were, two specks sitting motionlessly in a timeless summer sky.

The memory of that quiet, starless evening stayed in my mind like a lost photograph you discover in a pile of old letters and cannot stop staring at. How I wanted to go back to stop what had happened from happening!

I remembered the walk Jack and I had taken down a dirt road to an abandoned yellow house. "My dream house," I had told Jack as we stared at rambler rose and blackberry bushes gone so mad with growing that they had pushed their vines through windows and grew freely inside the house. "Dream house?" he said incredulously. "You're crazy. I want a place right on the beach with a big sun porch and an outdoor barbecue." Not me. I wanted a house with grass and trees and told him if he wanted his house on the beach he should move back to California. We argued, insulting each other's taste, and then laughed at how lucky we were not to have to make a decision because we couldn't afford to buy a house anyway.

I tried to hold on to the memory of that day, the way one tries to linger in the fantasy of a wonderful dream. But I could not pretend that all I remembered wasn't tainted with the ugly wounds of an accident, a stupid, pointless trick of nature. It was three o'clock in the morning by now, and Jack's parents had probably arrived at Kennedy Airport and would be at the house by six. I let my eyes close and told myself I had to sleep.

The last time I had seen Libbie and Lou was in Los Angeles at the tail end of our Mexican vacation. I'd been uncomfortable speaking to them long distance, but I discovered that being with them in their environment, lolling around the pool, wandering into the kitchen for a snack, was another story entirely. I began to relax with them and build a relationship based on a real affection for them rather than simply on my love for Jack, the one thing we all shared. When Jack spoke, I'd watch Lou's eyes. To say they filled up with love and admiration is corny, but that's just what I saw. He exuded pride. "I'm the father of that meshugana son-of-a-bitch," he'd say in a loud voice. Libbie reminded me of my own mother, except that she was more solicitous of me because I wasn't her daughter.

I heard the car on the gravel driveway and the doors slam shut. Another sunny day that hurt my eyes. I expected Lou to be crying and Libbie to be controlled. I ran downstairs and wrapped my arms around Libbie. She was sobbing, and we stood in the middle of the kitchen quietly cradling each other. I realized how much taller I was than she and that I wasn't crying. It was the first morning in days that I hadn't cried. When Libbie pulled away, she seemed a little embarrassed, but that didn't matter, and both she and I knew it. Then I saw Lou, who gave me a big hug and said, "Hiya, my little doll. It's going to be okay." I looked into his eyes—

round blue eyes with thick black lashes. He believed what he said. He wasn't crying. Sengstaken's words, "He will probably never walk again," no longer echoed in my head, but had been absorbed by my entire system, and I was just beginning to feel calm with the acceptance that Jack might not get better. And there was Lou standing in front of me, saying that everything was going to be okay. His optimism wasn't canned. He was scared, probably miserable, but he believed it—"Everything is going to be okay."

My mother went into the kitchen to fix coffee. She looked totally drained—her mouth was tense and she moved in jerks. I could tell that Lou made her nervous and that she felt on the verge of screaming. I followed her to the stove and put my arm around her. "Why don't you go inside and lie down?" I said.

"Don't be silly. I'm fine," she answered.

I noticed that she had sponged the same counter three times and washed the morning coffee cups twice instead of taking clean ones from the cupboard.

We moved out onto the porch, which was filled with sunlight. Libbie sat quietly on the swinging couch. She clutched a handkerchief with a big L embroidered on it and occasionally wiped her eyes behind the big light-blue sunglasses she was wearing.

Lou talked nervously. He didn't care what the doctors' prognoses were. Jack was going to pull through.

"I've seen Jack fight," he said. "I've seen him put his foot through a shower door in anger after he lost an important ball game. He'll play ball again. He won't give in. And we know a kid—you know, Libbie—who dove into a quarry and broke every bone in his body. He was paralyzed too. He's doing just great now. He was told he'd never walk again, too. But he's walking."

I could feel my mother's skin crawl, and I, too, wished that

Lou would shut up. The image of Jack kicking anything now, much less a shower door, was like a sick joke. The doctors said he wouldn't walk. How could Lou be so sure they were wrong? I tried to ignore what he was saying. I tried to remember what Joe had told me when I spoke to him after the operation. I'd called him before I went to sleep. I had asked him if Jack was better, and he said, "Mary. This is going to take a long time. If you go into the hospital every day expecting to see improvement, you'll go crazy. You can't expect any change, you can't expect anything."

I looked at Lou. He wasn't expecting anything. He knew. I wasn't angry with him but worried that his positiveness had nothing to do with reality, that if it was proved wrong, he'd be destroyed. I put the thought out of my head and said I was going upstairs to dress. Visiting hours weren't for two hours, but maybe they'd let us in early.

I tried to warn Libbie and Lou that Jack would be wired with tubes and tongs, but I knew nothing could soften the shock. I knocked on the windowless door of Intensive Care, and a stocky, round-faced nurse opened it a crack. I hated apologizing to everyone at the hospital, but in the early stages I always felt I was intruding. "I know we're here early," I said, "but Jack's parents just arrived from California." The nurse whispered that I should come in first and tell Jack they were here. I turned to Libbie and told her I'd be just a second and then she could go in. "IMMEDIATE FAMILY ONLY" was written in bold letters on the door. The words made me feel uncomfortable.

Jack's eyes were open, and the swelling had begun to go down. He tried to smile. I told him that his parents were here and wanted to see him. The tube in his nose made talking difficult, but he indicated that he was glad they were here. I kissed him gently on the forehead and said he shouldn't try to talk too much. We looked at each other for a

second longer, and then I realized I couldn't hog the brief
time allotted visitors.

Lou and I didn't speak as we waited for Libbie to come
out. We just looked at each other. Lou put his arm around
my shoulders, and I wrapped my arm around his waist. We
stood quietly together like two old friends who haven't seen
each other for years but whose physical proximity is a comforting proof that they share something very special. The
door opened, and as soon as Lou went in, Libbie embraced
me, crying, "My little baby, what have they done to my little
boy!" The reference to Jack as a baby confused me, all the
more because I was holding Libbie as one would a child. I
never once had thought of Jack as a little boy, even though
he was being cared for and had been robbed physically of
everything that made him a man. I realized that for Libbie
Jack would always be her "little boy," but the infantile reference annoyed me, seemed for an instant to threaten the intense attraction I still felt for him.

When Lou emerged from Intensive Care, his eyes
brimmed with tears, but he seemed almost buoyant. "I told
him that he's going to be all right," Lou said positively. "I
told him he had to fight, that he couldn't give in. I said we
were all with him and that he couldn't believe everything the
doctors said." Lou hesitated and looked at me. "I didn't say
that the doctors weren't good, but they're going to be wrong.
Look. I was told by some specialist son-of-a-bitch that I had
cancer. The schmuck sent the X-rays to the house by mistake
and I saw the diagnosis—carcinoma. He wanted to operate.
Well, I said, just wait a minute. You're not just going to cut
into me and mess around. I went to another doctor who
said, 'Lou, you're as healthy as an ox!' "

We walked toward the cafeteria, and I saw Joe Spinzia
approaching us briskly. He was in a hurry, and it seemed to
me that he really wanted to avoid us but knew he couldn't. I

introduced him to Libbie and Lou. He spoke quickly, as if speed would mitigate the horrible prognosis. I tried to steer him into an empty conference room or into a corner, but corridors have no corners and are not constructed for privacy. Somehow we managed to fall onto a green plastic couch, but Spinzia never sat down. He talked so quickly that Lou could hardly ask him a question, and then I realized that he was talking about hand surgery. "There are amazing things that can be done," he said. "Jack has some return in his flexors and extensors, so we could possibly transfer a muscle to his thumb. That way he could pinch. That's the most important function of the hand."

He talked almost compulsively, as though he didn't want to have to answer any questions. I couldn't slow him down, and I could tell that Libbie and Lou disliked him. I felt sorry for Joe because I could see that he couldn't deal with "the parents." He had been so direct and helpful to Jack and me, but this directness was just all wrong for Libbie and Lou. What is he trying to do? I thought to myself. Libbie and Lou have just arrived. They're tired and upset. Do they really want to be told about the miracles of hand surgery when they can see what terrible shape Jack's in now? I wished Joe would be gentler with them.

He excused himself to answer a phone call. Seconds later he told Lou that Sengstaken wanted to speak to him. "Dr. Sengstaken is more pessimistic than I," he said. "I still think there's a chance." I was glad he said that. I heard his voice soften and realized that he knew that he had been mishandling the situation but that he couldn't help it. Joe said he had to leave. "Maybe we can talk later," I said.

Lou walked toward us. He was pale and angry. "The son-of-a-bitch says the odds are ninety to ten against Jack's recovering. He's full of shit."

jack

The tube in my nose and throat made breathing difficult. I tried to disregard the discomfort and think about what Joe had said. I couldn't clear my mind. Paralysis, wheelchair, Mary, sex, marriage, children, job, friends, pity. I couldn't begin to deal with it. I sank deeper and deeper into mindless depression.

A pretty young nurse came over and tried to talk with me. We kidded about something. That was a little better. She even flirted a little, which made me feel better. She made me feel as if I were still a man. Then she disappeared. When she returned, she had a flower in a glass which she placed on the floor under my face. She told me she'd gone outside to pick it for me, but I figured she'd swiped it from another patient, probably someone who'd just died.

Over on my back again. Drugged, dozing, depressed. I sensed someone was there. I opened my eyes. It was Mary. We kissed. She seemed nervous and excited. We didn't talk about what we both knew. There was no time. She said my parents were outside, waiting to see me.

The night before, right before the operation, when Mary's father had asked me whether we should tell my parents to come, I'd wanted to say no. I had to go through this by myself, with Mary. I needed my strength and energy just to cope with my own situation. I was torn. I knew my parents had to be here. I wanted to see them but was afraid they might make things more difficult for me. I prepared myself to comfort *them*.

My mother came in first. She looked fine but controlled. She was wearing sunglasses so I couldn't tell what was going on inside her. I had no idea what I looked like to her, except that I knew I was still tan and thought that outwardly I looked pretty healthy. I could tell she didn't know how to start. She couldn't very well ask, "How are you?"

"How was the plane trip, Mom?"

"Oh, fine, a little tiring. But we're fine."

"And Dick. How are Dick and Cece?"

"They drove us to the airport. I think they'll be here soon. . . . Jack, do you hurt very badly?"

"No, Mom. I don't hurt. It was a freaky accident, but hell, I'm going to be okay. Don't worry. I'm just very tired, and it's hard to talk." She left and the nurse said how attractive she was.

Then, out of the corner of my eye, I saw my father. He was grinning, coming toward me with that crazy Groucho Marx lope of his, knees bent, arms swinging, skating across the floor. It was the same run, grin, and excitement he always had when he picked me up at the airport on my visits to Los Angeles. He'd shake my hand, throw his arm around my shoulders, and say, "Hiya, Jacko." He'd talk to me a mile a minute, never listening, while we picked up my bags and headed toward the car. Sometimes he'd be so excited that he couldn't find the car, and he'd usually lose his direction going home, even though he had been over the same route a hundred times.

Now he stood at my bed and grabbed my hand and said, "Hiya, Jacko." He didn't even give me a chance to say anything. "Listen, I don't care what the doctors or anyone else says. You'll beat it. You've been a scrapper all your life. You're the guy who breaks shower doors. You're a fighter, and no matter what else, you'll fight."

I tried to smile. I tried to answer, but I couldn't. He didn't ask me how I felt or how it happened or what I thought. Nothing. Just a few hours before, the doctor had told me I might not ever move again, and I knew that if my cord was torn, he was right. And here was this incredible man, happy to see me, telling me the doctors were full of shit and that he knew that I'd beat it. He wasn't telling me to be brave or to fight. He was telling me that he *knew* I'd fight.

I felt my eyes well up with tears. I was afraid to talk. I didn't want to break down in front of him. He started to leave.

"Dad . . . I'm glad you're here." I took a deep breath and began to choke up. "It means a lot to me . . . and I'll fight."

"I know you will," he said and left. I broke down and cried.

That night they rolled me out of Intensive Care and back to my room. My brother, Dick, and his wife, Cece, were there. I was happy to see them.

It didn't occur to me until later that the family suddenly being there meant I could have died. I never thought of it—it just seemed natural for them to be here now.

Dick is four years younger than I and was a dentist who worked in the Watts Clinic in L.A. We had always been very close as kids, and even though we lived at opposite ends of the country, we remained close. I was also crazy about Cece, who was pretty, warm, and open.

"Hey, how'd you get away from work?" I said.

"I'm not working this summer," Cece said in her soft voice. She was a teacher.

"And I just left," Dick said, flashing me that big toothy grin of his. We both wore braces when we were kids and picked up the habit of lifting our upper lip, all the way to the gums, when we smiled, so as not to get ourselves hooked onto the wires.

"Actually, I took a short leave of absence," he said.

Mary had first met Dick, Cece, and my parents when we'd spent Thanksgiving in L.A. our first year together. I had been raised there but left for New York after I got out of school. I left L.A. because I didn't like it. I still don't like it. But being there with Mary was different. I got a kick out of showing her around and trying to explain what it was like growing up there. She humbly suggested that we make a movie about our trip called "Mary Goes to California," starring Mary Pleshette. She loved it. She'd never seen anything like it before. We stayed with Dick and Cece in their old frame house in Santa Monica, just half a block from the beach. The area used to house Midwesterners who had come out to California to retire, or, as the local joke went, where old folks came to visit their parents. Now it was a nice little community of working-class people and a lot of young kids.

We spent time with my folks but mostly with Dick and Cece. The weather was beautiful, and we went to the beach. Mary couldn't get over the fact that it was Thanksgiving and warm enough to swim. We drove through Beverly Hills and Brentwood. We looked at movie stars' homes and saw L.A. at night from the hills. We tried to stand in the footprints of the famous at Grauman's Chinese, and we shopped at boutiques and stared at freaks on Hollywood Boulevard.

But most of all we ate. The Pleshettes pride themselves on loving to eat, especially fine food. John's a gourmet cook. Norman has his Nova sent from Scotland and his mints from London. Mary claims tears came to her eyes when she ate fresh raspberries at a famous restaurant in the South of France and that five years later she could still remember every meal she ate there. But in L.A., as far as I'm concerned, *haute cuisine* is hamburgers and hot dogs. So, with Dick and Cece, both connoisseurs, we hit every three-star stand in town. For breakfast it was Hamburger Square in Venice, for lunch Hamburger Hamlet, and for dinner Pinks.

Now, in the hospital, we were all back together again. Dick and I stared at each other for a long time. Mary and Cece stood a little behind. I wondered what I must look like to Dick and what was going through his mind. I knew that with his medical training he probably understood a lot about what was happening to me, but I didn't want to ask. I was too scared. I wanted to joke but couldn't. He looked too serious and upset. He didn't feel the need to say or do or offer anything. I had the feeling he knew exactly what I was feeling and that a part of him was attached to the tongs with me. "It took less than a second to change my life," I said, breaking the silence. Dick just nodded.

The fourth night in the hospital I had nightmares again. This time I dreamed of the wave, tumbling over and over, falling and smashing my head on the sand. I could feel my head jerk and the horrible spasms in my neck and back. I woke up scared. I thought I had lifted out of the tongs, but I hadn't. That was impossible. I closed my eyes and went back to sleep and had the same dream, falling, falling, crashing down, and the pain. It was like diving into an empty swimming pool.

I awoke and called for the nurse. Like a kid scared of the dark, I asked her to turn on the light. She said the dreams might be caused by the Demerol. Then she turned me on my stomach, and for the first time I relaxed in that position. I let my arms hang down and asked one of the aides if she had time to give me a massage. Her hands kneaded my shoulders and back muscles. I lay there staring down at the floor, the straps supporting my head. I didn't think of anything. I just let myself feel her hands. The fear caused by the dreams slowly disappeared. The nightmares had been so terrifying, and I'd been so relieved when the nurse came in and turned on the light that I realized that I'd lost my fear of being turned over onto my stomach. I didn't notice the straps cutting into my forehead and chin. I just went limp, exhausted from the night, and stared mindlessly down at the floor.

I felt more relaxed after she turned me back. "I'm better. You can turn off the lights," I said.

"It's okay," she said, as if I were a little boy scared of the dark. "The sun is coming up."

She was right. I did feel safer with the dawn.

"You know, it's time for your shot," she said. "Do you think you can take it?"

"I think so. I'm okay."

This time I dreamed I was running. I tripped and fell forward, my neck jerked, and the pain woke me up. Afraid to close my eyes, I lay there staring at the ceiling, fighting off the drug, wanting to close my eyes, afraid to, waiting for it to wear off.

When Joe came in later that day, I told him about my bad trips.

"Sometimes Demerol can do that," he said. "We'll try another drug. Also, I think I'm going to change your roommate."

"Why?"

"Well, there's a young kid down the hall who'll be better company for you. The old man is out of it too much of the time, and I think you'll like this other guy. You'll be good for each other."

"It's okay with me. . . . Too bad I never found out where the old man hid his loot."

My room was so small that they had to maneuver my bed around into a corner in order to get my old roommate out and my new roommate in. Out of the corner of my eye I saw someone being rolled in. Rather, I saw an arm and leg in a cast suspended from a metal frame above his bed. Because I couldn't see the bed itself, he appeared to be hanging like a chimpanzee in the zoo. "Hi," I said. "Welcome."

"Hi," he said as they wheeled him past me, "I hear you're in really shitty shape. . . . Hey, sweetheart, Patti," he called to a nurse as soon as his bed was in place. "Where is my table and the radio? And be careful when you bring it in. My cigarettes and watch are in the drawer, and don't forget my Bermuda shorts, the checked ones, and my shirts." Then he turned his attention to me. "Hi. I'm Mike Guerin."

"Hi. I'm Jack Willis. Where you from?"

"The Bronx."

I had guessed from his voice that he was around thirty years old. In a second the nurse was back with an armful.

"Hang them up neatly," he ordered. "No. Don't put the table there, dummy. How can I reach it? Put it on my left side with the drawer facing me. That's a good girl. Now light me a cigarette, will you? And I'm expecting a phone call from my lawyer, so will you listen and grab the phone for me if it rings?"

Then he said, "Hey, Jack, man, what happened to you?"

"I was flipped by a wave and broke my neck."

"Wow." He half laughed. "Ain't that a pisser? The surf did all that to you. Man, I've never heard of *anyone* getting his neck broke by a wave."

"Me either," I said. "What happened to you?"

"It's crazy, man. We got this place in Hampton Bays, lots of girls, guys, always something doing. Three weeks ago my buddy and I went out for dinner and some fun. We were driving home when I saw this guy step out into the road. My buddy swerved, and that's the last thing I remember."

"You were in a coma," I said.

"A coma? Man, I didn't wake up till ten days later. I think we went off an embankment and I was thrown out of the car. And then the car rolled over onto me. They told me that when they found me, I had so little pulse they gave me the last rites."

"What happened to your friend?"

"Nothing, man. Do you believe it? He walked away without a scratch, the bastard. All he lost was his car. And I've been here three weeks.

"The nurses say those first ten days I was out of my mind. They say I'd have clear conversations and then I'd start swearing and screaming. I don't remember a thing. I've been here three weeks now, the longest of any patient on Surgical One. Doctors say I'll be here another three to four months with this arm and leg of mine all busted up. My mother was with me those first few days. She says I was crazy. I don't even remember her being here. Same with my girl friend, Muggs—Valerie is her real name, but I call her Muggs. She's not really my girl—I mean I like her, but I don't want to settle down now. She's only one of my girl friends, but don't tell her. Anyway, she says I tore up my bandages and swore at the nurses. I even tried to tear out the tubes they had running through me. I don't remember." Mike paused for just a second. "Hey, sweetheart," he yelled into the hall, "can you turn the TV around so I can see it? What the hell good is it doing facing the door?"

Early the next day, when they gave me a shot and turned me onto my stomach, Mike offered me his radio.

"Hey, sweetheart, put it down by his head so he can hear. What d'ya like, Jack?"

"It's okay, Mike," I said. "You keep it. I'll just sleep."

"No. You take it," he said, and made sure the nurses put it on the floor a few feet from my head. "Hey, sweetheart," Mike said, "turn it up, will you, so I can hear it too?"

A nurse came over to my bed and gave me a shot. I closed my eyes, tired from a sleepless night, and gave in to the drug. The music from Mike's radio was blasting, but I didn't want to hurt his feelings by asking him to turn it down. I lay there, torn between telling him to turn the damn thing off and just letting it blare. Then the drug began to work, and I was somewhere between a world of sleep and a world of complete lucidity. Colors, bright and beautiful colors, filled my head. I began to hear the music, and the colors danced, changed, and flashed to the rock beat. I gave in and went with it. Part of me watched while the other part fixed on the beat and moved with the rhythms. I forgot the discomfort of the straps across my forehead and chin.

When they turned me onto my back, the white hospital ceiling was a rich blue. I forgot the music and watched the paint move across the ceiling. The texture and color looked like paint when you mix it in its can before it is completely blended. Mary, Dick, and Cece came into the room and I started to tell them about what I saw. But then they began to close in on me. My brother's smile and the look of concern in Mary's eyes made me nervous, and I closed my eyes tight, trying to stop the drug. Finally my head stopped spinning and the colors disappeared, so I opened my eyes. I looked up at the ceiling; the paint was still a rippling blue. Everyone was moving in on me, coming closer and closer to my head. I tried to explain what was happening, but I was getting more and more nervous and out of control. I asked them all to leave.

When I told Joe what had happened to me, he very cautiously asked me what my past drug experience had been. I guess he thought I was part of some wild New York scene. "Almost nothing," I said. "A little social smoking, some pot— you know. Why?"

"Because if you'd been a heavy user that might explain your extraordinary reaction to what is usually a harmless drug."

"Well, I'm not a heavy user," I said. I wasn't sure whether I convinced him of that, but he decided to give me morphine. At first I felt nothing. Then I felt a warmth, beginning in my legs, that slowly crept upward, enveloping my entire body. I felt as if I were slipping slowly into a warm tub of water. I felt myself drifting, slowly drifting off, feeling warm, comfortable, and safe.

Dick, Cece, and I went into the conference room across the hall from Jack's room. The bright lights bounced off the flat yellow walls, making all our skin look a sickly jaundice color. I looked out the screened window into a black night and could hear the sprinklers click as they made their full circle of watering the hospital lawn. For some reason the sound irritated me, but I was too tired to care. I wanted Spinzia to talk with Dick. I wanted Dick to understand so he could explain to Libbie and Lou. And, I didn't know why, but I wanted to hear it all again. Maybe I still didn't believe it myself.

Spinzia came into the room and sat down. He was tense, but acted casual, as if he'd already done the explaining routine and would waste no time getting into hard facts. "Have you thought about a rehab hospital?" he said, and seeing the look of dismay on our faces, he went right on. "I know you're shaking your heads. But Jack is going to need a lot of care. And that care costs a lot of money. You can't just put it off."

I was struck by the notion that Joe was talking about someone else, discussing the fate of a faceless cripple. Dick slumped in his chair, but his words came quickly, without hesitation.

"Before we talk about rehabilitation, I want to know why you say you're more optimistic than Sengstaken."

"I don't think Jack's cord was severed. I think there's a chance it was badly bruised. If I'm right, he'll get return in around two to three weeks."

I looked at Dick. "Sengstaken says the odds are only ten per cent, but if Jack's that ten per cent, it's a hundred for us," Dick said. Cece and I smiled.

"We never know with these spinal injuries," Joe said. "There can be complications." Joe paused. "I just want you to know that I think Jack is an incredible man. I could never go through what he's going through. Maybe I shouldn't say that, but I'm the kind of guy who gets all his relaxation from working with his hands. When I go home, I work on old cars. I get them when they're piles of junk and transform them into collectors' items. Even if Jack gets some return, the chances are slim that he'll be able to use his hands. Luckily, there is surgery that can be performed that would restore some movement in that area."

I wasn't listening. "Complications? What kind of complications?" I blurted out.

"I guess the most dangerous is pneumonia. If a quadriplegic begins to collect fluid in his lungs, he has no way of getting it out because he doesn't have the muscles to cough. And then there's the catheter. . . . If it stays in too long, he could develop strictures which would cut off his ability to urinate . . ."

"And ejaculate," I interrupted. The fear of pneumonia didn't frighten me, but the mention of strictures in his penis terrified me. I wished Joe hadn't mentioned them. He had told me too much already. Why did he have to mention strictures?

"How long can the catheter stay in before it's dangerous?" I asked.

"A pretty long time," he said, trying to be understanding. "That's the least of my worries. We can always catheterize him by inserting a tube right into the bladder, a supra-pubic catheterization."

I pretended to be relieved, but I could hear myself crying inside, "Strictures. Oh, God, please don't let that happen!"

Dick asked a few more questions, and then Joe got up to leave.

"Do you have any children?" I asked.

"Yes. Two girls."

I had stopped taking The Pill the morning after the operation. I felt a little like a novice whose outer vestments and gold wedding band are as much a symbol of abstinence as a protection against any lingering desire to sin. There seemed no point to protecting myself. My sex life had been washed out to sea with that wave, and the strange part of it all was that I felt no frustration, no physical withdrawal. If I thought of Jack's and my lovemaking, I felt a deep sadness, an empty, hollow nostalgia, but I had lost touch with my sexuality. And in a peculiar way, sex seemed irrelevant. The closeness was still there, the warmth; the need to share was now satisfied by a look, a touch, a kiss.

I had always imagined that the day I would decide not to take The Pill would be a happy day, a secret, joyous day. I wouldn't tell anyone that I was trying to get pregnant, but I'd know and Jack would know. . . . And when it happened, we'd surprise everyone the same way we had surprised them about our wedding. I looked at the half-empty packet of pills. The little white "Tuesday" pill was neatly protected by plastic. Just a week before, I would have reacted immediately, a little panicked, "Oh, Christ, I forgot to take my pill," but now I just stared back at the purplish-pink case. I clicked the remaining pills out into the palm of my hand and threw them into the toilet bowl.

I felt defiant and angry, more anxious to get pregnant now than ever before. We would have a child as soon as we could. Sengstaken said we could still do that. "I'll show them," I said to myself. "I'll show them and get pregnant right away." I fantasized walking into Sengstaken's office one day, big-bellied and glowing. I even imagined Jack playing with a baby. The thought of his not being able to run or play with a child didn't frighten me. I tried to picture him in a wheelchair, surrounded by a family, our family. I focused on this idealized vision the way one looks at a collage, not con-

centrating on the individual parts of the painting but looking at the work as a whole. I didn't think about details, I
didn't dissect the elements. I couldn't imagine what life
would be with a man in a wheelchair—the ramps, the special
bars and equipment for bathrooms and halls. I didn't try to
imagine how we would have sex. "We will do it," I said to
myself. "Somehow we will make it work."

My great desire to have a child or, really, to be pregnant,
was totally illogical, but my life seemed to have no relation to
logic, no connection to rational planning. I felt removed
from the neat schedules of *Newsweek,* from the normal
schemes which had marked the days and months and years
of my previous life. I had been left on an island with no
clocks or calendars and had only the rhythms of nature to
tell me that time had passed, was passing. I felt stripped of
expectancy, and the future didn't seem to matter. I felt
strangely natural, unprotected, yet strong. Having a baby
somehow echoed my feelings of "naturalness." My life was
comprised of basics—all the frills and fancies were now
clean, straight lines. And having a baby seemed as basic as
anything could be. I didn't think that my womanliness had
been taken away from me, but that's what I must have felt. I
tried not to think about Jack's touching my body, making me
feel myself through his love and appreciation. I didn't think
about what I was missing, but I still missed it. Having a baby
seemed a beautiful metaphor for feeling life, giving life,
being totally, physically alive.

jack

Like a baby, I was totally dependent upon others for everything. I had to be fed, cleaned, made comfortable. I had no control over my bladder, and defecation was induced. Unlike a baby, I had the brain of a man and the memory of what I had been and also the understanding of what I might be.

I tried to scratch my nose, but like a spastic, I missed it completely. When I got close to it, I couldn't use my fingers. It felt more natural for me to scratch with the heel of my hand. I knew Mary was watching, and I wondered what she was thinking. Maybe, like me, she was remembering all those jokes we used to tell about spastics, like the boy who misses his mouth and hits himself in the forehead with an ice-cream cone. I tried not to think about the jokes. I even felt a funny kind of pride in just getting my hand close to my face, and I wondered why I hadn't tried to do it before.

When lunch was brought to me, I asked Mary to place my sandwich in my hand so I could try to feed myself. They had taken me off intravenous feeding two days before, and since then either Clive or Mary had fed me. Now she placed the sandwich between my forefinger and thumb, but if fell out. I couldn't hold it. "Try again," I barked. I got a better grip and started to move it toward my mouth, fighting gravity. The ham and cheese started to slip out. It didn't occur to me to use my other hand to help. I rushed the whole thing toward my mouth, but all the ham and cheese fell onto my chest; like the kid with the ice-cream cone, I hit myself in the cheek with the bread.

After a couple of tries I got a small bite. I was sweating, and the effort exhausted me. But I started thinking ahead to the next meal and for a moment forgot that the rest of me was paralyzed.

I tried to concentrate on other things I could do. There was a little stand attached to the underside of my bed. I

thought maybe I could read, and I asked Clive to get me a
newspaper and lay it flat below me. I tried to turn the pages,
but my hands were useless, paralyzed and numb. I discovered that if I bent my wrist backward, I could open my forefinger and thumb and that if I bent my wrist forward, I
could force the fingers into something resembling a pinch. I
tried turning the pages that way, but because my fingers
were numb, I couldn't feel the paper. The head nurse, Janet
LaVinio, suggested I use the heel of my hand to push the
page and crumple it. Then I could dog-ear the bottom of
the paper and would have something to pinch. That way,
maybe, I could turn it. It took me forty-five minutes to read
a quarter of the *Times*. Janet stayed with me and massaged
my back and shoulders. She brought me some juice in a cup
and, exhausted, I waited for her to feed it to me.

"Try it yourself," she said and placed a straw in the cup.

I tried gripping the cup between my hands. But it was
heavy to lift, and I couldn't co-ordinate lifting the cup and
placing the straw between my lips. So I picked up the straw,
put that into my mouth first, then lifted the cup around the
straw. When the cup was half full, it was finally light enough
for me to handle, straw and all. When it was empty, I put it
down on the stand, both elated and depressed by my accomplishment. I thought about how weak and unco-or-
dinated my arms were and they weren't even paralyzed. I
wondered how weak the rest of my body would be, even if I
got return.

That night after all the visitors had gone, Joe dropped in
to say hello. He had come to the hospital to check another
patient. Now that he was finished, he was relaxing, his foot
propped up on the chair next to my bed, puffing on a cigar.
We made small talk for a while. I could tell he wanted to stay
and talk but didn't know quite how to do it. I sensed he was
afraid to get too close to me, afraid of straining what he

thought was the doctor-patient relationship. But that's exactly what I wanted. I wanted to get as close to the guy as possible. I needed continual reassurance that he really cared for me. To do that, he had to understand me. So what I really wanted to talk about was me, but because he was unsure of himself, I knew to keep him there we'd have to talk about him.

"Pretty tough racket?" I began.

"Yeah. But I love it. The hours don't bother me, and I'm really my own man."

"What do you mean? You're here all day and night."

"Sure," he said defensively, "but I get time off. I live only five minutes from the hospital, and my office is right across the road. I work hard, but I can run home and see my kids. If patients get on my nerves, I can just knock off work a few days." He shifted his legs on the chair, unwinding a little more.

"Baloney," I said. "I've seen you here over the weekend and almost every night. It's not as good as you make it sound. You don't relax."

"Well, summer's the big season around here—all you dumb city folk come out here, run around and get hurt—auto accidents, swimming accidents. Weekends we get 'em piled up in the halls. But winter's soft. I get to work on my car."

"Car?"

"Yeah. I rebuild old cars. Buy them cheap and rebuild them. I like working with my hands . . . be a lot tougher on me if I was in your position."

I heard my voice rise. "What do you mean by that?"

"In my work I depend on my hands. You work with your head."

"Yeah, well, I also work with my hands and legs."

"But it'd be tougher for me to adjust."

"Bullshit. What do you think I'm going to do if I'm stuck in a wheelchair the rest of my life? I wasn't sitting on my ass—I made films, and I love sports, and what about a family?"

"Well, sports aren't important," Joe interrupted.

"Maybe not to you, but . . ."

"And maybe you can still have a family."

"Maybe. Maybe," I said, but felt depressed. He wasn't giving one inch. He wasn't telling me anything he hadn't told me before. I tried to shift gears. "Have you had other broken necks here?"

"No broken necks, but a couple of years ago we had a young guy who broke his back in an auto accident and was paralyzed from the waist down. He's still in a wheelchair, but he drives a car—hand controls."

Big deal, I thought. He thinks the worst thing about paralysis is not being able to drive a car. Nothing about not having control over your bladder and bowels or not being able to fuck or run or work. "Is he married?" I asked.

"Yeah. He has a wife. I'm not sure about kids."

"Last night I asked the evening nurse about other patients. I ask everybody, nurses, aides, even the cleaning lady. . . ."

Joe laughed.

"And Phyllis said that usually when there's feeling there's motor control and that eventually there's return. And I have feeling. I can feel texture like my top sheet or the sheepskins or the pressure of a hand, even though I can't feel pain or hot and cold." I wanted Joe to tell me that Phyllis was right—I'd get back control.

"Every patient asks the same questions," he said. "But there are no rules. Each case is entirely different, and just because some guy had the same symptoms and recovered doesn't mean that it'll be the same for you."

After he left, I thought about what he'd said, how it would have been more difficult for him than it was for me because he worked with his hands. I dropped that sandwich because I couldn't pinch. I could only manipulate my thumb and forefinger a little by bending my wrist. And even then I couldn't exert enough pressure to prevent it from falling out of my hands. I dropped it because my hands were numb and felt as though they had gone to sleep. That's the way the rest of my body felt—asleep.

I thought of my numb hands. I thought of trying to caress Mary or to type a letter or to play catch or to carry an envelope home from work. I didn't want to be like a baby, dependent on others. I thought of how unfair it was, especially for Mary, that I was racked up like this. But, strangely, I didn't feel a need to talk with her about it because I knew her well enough to know that she would be totally honest with me and with herself. If she was with me, it was because she wanted to be with me, because she still loved me, not because she felt pity for me or had some misplaced sense of duty. And I also knew that when she felt that she could no longer stand it or that she didn't love me, she would leave. But for the moment I was confident—confident of the fight in her and of the love we shared.

I fell into a half sleep. I dreamed I was holding Mary. It was more than a dream. It was so real I could actually feel her. She was in bed with me. I was in a half-sitting position and she was lying against my shoulder. We kissed. I touched her. I could smell her hair and body. I could feel her softness as I stroked her hair. Her skin was wet and the odors of our sweat commingled in the hot room. We kissed some more, and I held her closely and stroked her head. I kept telling her that everything was going to be okay and she believed me. We both believed it.

I woke up drenched in sweat. I was alone except for Mike

in the next bed. I began thinking about all the good times Mary and I had had. I began thinking about the unfairness of the accident. I tried to imagine not taking that wave. I imagined myself diving under it and the two of us coming out of the water together, going home to a barbecue dinner. We would have sat outdoors and watched the sun set, and maybe that night after dinner we would have gone down to the beach to lie in the sand and stare at the stars.

During the past week or so I would have worked on the new show. I knew from my secretary, who'd come out to visit, that it wasn't going well. I'd had a lot of ideas that I thought would help make it work. But now I didn't care. Now it was the weekend, and if I hadn't taken that wave, we'd be back out there at the beach. I would have gotten up and gone to town to buy a newspaper and whatever we needed for breakfast. Then I would have gone to the beach and jogged along the hard sand at the water's edge. It was a hot morning, and the sweat would have come easily, but the ocean breeze would have evaporated it almost immediately. If it was really hot, I would have gone into the ocean for a short swim, and then I would have gone back to the house to wake Mary to have some breakfast together before heading for a day on the beach.

But I wasn't having breakfast with Mary. I was staring up at the perforated tiles on the ceiling above my head in the Southampton hospital. I was lying there sweating my ass off, waiting for the morning shift to come on, for a new hospital day to begin, for somebody to feed me my breakfast. I really was like a baby. If there was no return, I'd probably need a full-time nurse to care for me. And where I had been confident just half an hour before of Mary's and my love, I now couldn't imagine her staying with me. I couldn't imagine her changing the catheter, giving me suppositories, pushing me around in a wheelchair. I knew that some people did it. But

I couldn't imagine our doing it. If the roles had been reversed, I couldn't have done it, and I didn't want her to. She was young, healthy, and alive. If I were in a wheelchair, I couldn't see how I could satisfy any of her needs.

I thought of the future and of being alone. Maybe I could teach, not in New York—how could I get around the city in a wheelchair? Maybe the University of Miami, or somewhere in California—Pomona or Mills. I pictured the campus and being pushed to class and home again. I thought of what Joe and the nurses said about the spinal-injury cases they knew. "Why, he can even drive a car. You know, hand controls." So I pictured myself driving, lifting myself up out of the car, being pushed up and down special ramps.

I remembered a guy in college who was in a wheelchair and managed to push himself around. He could even get up and down curbs by tipping the chair backward until the two tiny front wheels were on the curb and then forcing the back wheels up and over. He was big and good-looking, very strong through the chest and shoulders.

I saw myself in a chair like him, withered legs and disproportionately large chest and shoulder muscles. I had had a couple of classes with him. He was bright and lively and appeared to have a lot of friends. But who knew what went through his mind when he was alone? Did he brood as I did about the past? Did he have any meaningful relationships with women? Did he have sex? Did he have the same dark thoughts I had now when he thought about the future?

I didn't know how he'd been hurt. But now I wished I'd taken the time to talk with him—not for him, but for me. Maybe I'd have a better idea of what it was going to be like. I wondered what he was doing and if he was happy. I thought about teaching again and knew I didn't want to do that. It sounded awfully dull after making films. But what else could I do? I tried not to think about it. I tried to fall asleep.

mary

I watched Jack sleep. The blood around the tongs was dry and black, and the hair around his ears was already beginning to grow back. His lips had a sticky film over them, and he smelled of sleep. His eyes fluttered lightly, and I wondered what he was dreaming. I looked over his body, big and silent, and tried to convince myself that he really couldn't move. I pinched his thigh, secretly hoping that it would twitch or slide away from my touch. But it stayed in place, heavy and dead. I imagined that I was looking at a corpse, not Jack, but a stranger. His chest didn't move with breathing, and his mouth was slightly open, the corners cracked and dry.

I longed for the time when Jack and I would be in control of our lives without the advice or hopes of all those who now surrounded us. I thought of suicide, of helping Jack kill himself. I wondered how we'd do it. Then I thought what if it had been the other way around. Maybe it would have been better, at least easier. I remembered the slow, measured words of Sengstaken when I asked him if Jack and I would be able to make love. "Jack will be able to get some kind of erection, but he won't feel anything. . . . You will have to be the active partner." What about children, could we still have children? "Yes, he could still ejaculate. Many paraplegics have children. . . ." The words rushed in front of my eyes like ticker tape. The memory of that first mention of "paraplegic" and the sickening effect it had had on me returned. If I had been the one, if I were paralyzed, I could still be made love to. I could still have a baby. I couldn't feel, but . . . I didn't know. The thoughts flooded my mind, mixed-up thoughts, thoughts that frightened me. I wouldn't be able to dance, to run. My legs would wither, and I wouldn't be able to wear pretty sandals or short skirts. But the worst, the very worst would have been their shaving off my hair. I didn't think about the pain of having holes drilled into my head. All cosmetic, all vanity.

I stopped projecting. It hadn't happened to me. It had happened to a part of me, to the one person from whom I didn't want to separate myself. I wondered why the same thoughts didn't frighten me when I realized it *was* happening to Jack. I didn't project about us. I knew from the moment I said I wanted Jack to live that the future couldn't be tampered with, that what lay ahead nobody could know. Jack opened his eyes and ran his tongue over his mouth. It almost seemed a miracle that he was alive, that he was not a stranger.

Jack smiled at me, and for a moment I was reminded of the lazy, happy smiles that spread with yawns over our faces when we used to wake up together in the same bed.

"How you feeling, baby?" he said. "Come here and kiss me."

We kissed and I could tell that Jack was beginning to smell like the clean but stagnant air of the hospital. There was no odor of sweat, no smell of dirt, no overpowering scent of perfumed disinfectant. Just a different smell, one of inactivity, of no sun and no fresh air.

"How did you sleep?" I asked.

"Okay. I had some bad dreams, but I slept soundly from around five till eight. . . . What about you?"

"Pretty well, I guess. I don't have sleep problems. It's just strange sleeping alone. . . . Oh, Jack, I miss you so." I rested my head on his chest and closed my eyes. I felt him rub his arms over my hair. We didn't speak, and I wanted to crawl up onto that skinny frame and lie down with him.

"Time for your pills, Mr. Willis," a pimply-faced nurse with a twangy Midwestern voice said gaily. "Now, you get the yellow one, two whites, and an orange. There we go," she said, bending the straw into Jack's mouth. Her harlequin glasses began to slide down her long, pointy nose. Somehow, with both her hands full, she managed quite deftly to push them back in place. "How we doin' today, Jack?" And as soon as Jack said, "Fine," she was off with a squeak of her rubber-soled shoes to dispense pills to somebody else. Then a mousy girl in a pink nurse's aide uniform wheeled in a tray filled with aluminum-covered dishes. I timidly removed a sweaty cover and stared at Jack's lunch—a ham-and-cheese sandwich on Tip-Top Bread, suffocated by steam. Off came another cover—iceberg lettuce, topped with some tired slices of tomato, the whole salad limp and lukewarm. Dessert was a piece of cake and some Del Monte pears. Every meal began with a large glass of cranberry juice, which cleaned out Jack's kidneys and staved off infection. I broke the sandwich into quarters and began feeding it to Jack. The salad, dripping with neon-orange dressing, required more care. I had to cup one hand under the other to avoid splattering Jack's face with the sticky liquid. At one point, a precariously balanced piece of tomato fell somewhere between his mouth and cheekbone. Jack and I began to laugh. The whole operation seemed so ridiculous that neither of us could have stood it without laughing.

Jack was usually turned onto his stomach shortly after lunch. I was just beginning to be able to bear looking at this procedure without feeling panic or nausea. I knew how painful it had been a week before, and the sound of Jack's cries made me shiver with fear and anger and frustration because I knew there was nothing I could do to stop it. Now he gave the nurses instructions, and they did their best to follow them.

"Strap me in tighter," Jack said. "That's it. Can't you put something, maybe a piece of sheepskin or something, between my chin and the strap? Great. That's fine. Okay, I'm ready."

Squashed between the sheepskins, metal frame, and straps, Jack looked like a grotesque human sandwich. The moment they turned him, I froze. Reflexively I waited for him to cry out in pain, even though he hadn't for almost a week. As he lay on his stomach, Jack's back still looked muscular and tan. A bandage covered the incision which ran almost seven inches from the nape of his neck down his back. I'd expected a much larger bandage and a meaner-looking scar, but the surgeons cut into Jack with such artistry that the skin was healing perfectly and it looked as if someone had taken a delicate brush and painted a straight line down the center of his back.

I sat down in the corner, hardly roomy enough for a chair, picked up the *Times,* and started reading aloud. I felt so far away from the news, so distant from the rest of the world. I looked over to Jack and put my hand on his arm. His skin was warm, and as I touched him, I felt a wave of love wash over me. I felt strangely at peace, settled, almost cozy. Jack may have been waiting for signs of change, secret signals of improvement, but I didn't dare wait. I had expected to be married in the fall, to be pregnant by spring, to live happily ever after. Now I was wary of expectation; I mistrusted the future . . . or maybe I was simply terrified of more disappointment.

Jack had fallen asleep again. I watched his belly rise and fall with the quiet rhythms of sleep. He lay perfectly still, never twitched or jerked. It was as if his dreams were tied down by the same invisible net that immobilized his body. At times I felt I was guarding him, protecting him from noise and sudden awakening. I'd look at his body and wonder if he'd ever move again. What does it feel like to be paralyzed, I thought in the silence of that muggy room. I tried to keep my hand in one position and pick up a paper cup. Like Jack,

I'd bend my wrist to open my fingers and then bend it back to tighten my hold. But there was no way I could know or understand or feel what Jack was going through. As I started to lift the cup, I invariably felt the muscles in my fingers grip the cup in complete defiance of my simulated paralysis. With the tiniest effort, I would crush the cup with one hand into a waxy ball and throw it into a trash basket on the other side of the room.

The Willises had finally moved into a house of their own. For the first emergency nights both families had lived together; Libbie and Lou slept upstairs, as did Dick and Cece. I slept with my mother after my father returned to New York, and John slept on the living-room floor. We were still eating numerous meals together, but even that was difficult. The accident had pulled everyone together, but we couldn't really feel close. It was as if we had been lassoed and were beginning to feel the burn of the rope. There was a growing need for privacy, for being able to grieve with our own clan.

It was the first meal in a week that the two families hadn't been together. I stared at the food in front of me. My mother had done all the work, and I'd been called to the table from a nap upstairs. The drumstick lying dead on my plate seemed to be daring me to eat it, and the pleasure of eating was now just a necessary function. "You have to eat something," my mother said. "You need your strength."

My strength. Getting through the meal seemed an extraordinary effort. I managed to finish the chicken and a few teaspoons of rice, and though I could feel the food land hard somewhere in my stomach, I felt I had eaten nothing. At one point during the meal I realized that my eyes were riveted on the chicken neck which someone had picked clean. I could see the vertebrae and the exposed slippery cord that ran through it. So that's what it looks like a little.

The connection both revolted and fascinated me. Someone whisked the plate away, and the trance was broken.

After the dishes were washed (I was excused from that task, too), I walked into the bedroom that had been Jack's and mine just a while before. I climbed up on the bed, which faced a long mirror, and stared at my image, no longer comforted by my lingering suntan, but cynically amused by my loneliness. "What a waste," I said to myself. "I thought I'd finally made it. I'd found the right guy."

Mama came into the room and immediately looked to see if I was crying. She sat down on the bed and took my hand. Before she could say anything and despite her efforts to hold back the tears, she started to weep. She tried to stifle her sobs with a Kleenex she had pulled from the sleeve of her sweater, but she was too exhausted to control herself, and I wished she would stop trying to be so strong. "Cry, Mama, go ahead. Let it all out," I said, wrapping my arms around her.

"It's so unfair." She shook her head. "You're so young and beautiful. . . ." And then she stopped herself, embarrassed to say what was really on her mind. She took a deep breath. "I shouldn't be crying. I'm your mother. I should be comforting you."

"But you are comforting me. Don't hold back. Talk it out. Then you'll feel better."

My coaxing seemed to work, and Mama let herself cry freely. For a moment I realized we were more than a mother and daughter grieving together. We were two women who understood each other because we knew what it was to love a man so deeply.

"I guess it upsets me so to see you hurt because I know how hard it is," she said. "There was a time in my marriage when Papa was sick and we were pretty miserable." She hesitated. "I guess if I hadn't loved him so much, I wouldn't

have been able to stay with him. But the one thing a mother
hopes is that her children will be spared that pain. . . ."
She began to cry again. "I just hate to see you go through
this. You shouldn't have to deal with these problems now."
"I know I shouldn't. But I have no choice, just as you had
no choice. Just understand that I love Jack and that he loves
me. We still don't know what's going to happen."
Mama looked at me and tried to brace herself against
more tears. "If Jack doesn't improve, he won't want you
to . . ." She stopped.
"To marry him," I finished her sentence. "We're not there
yet, Mama. We don't have to decide anything now."
I could see she felt guilty for thinking she *hoped* he
wouldn't marry me, even though she never said it out loud.
But I wasn't angry with her, and I didn't have to say that the
decision to get married would be Jack's and mine, would
have nothing to do with her hopes or fears. "Do you feel better?" I said.
Mama suddenly seemed to remember she was a mother.
"I'm fine. Now you get into bed and get some rest. You can't
let yourself get exhausted. And you're getting too thin. Your
face looks pinched." I climbed into bed and let her tuck me
in. She kissed me good night, but before she left she said:
"You're a wonderful girl, Mary. I love you very much."

The next day I hesitated before entering Jack's room. At
first I thought he was asleep, but then I saw that his eyes
were open and that he was staring at the ceiling.
I walked over to his bed and kissed him. His eyes looked
cloudy and his mouth was grimly set. I put my hand on his
forehead. "What's the matter, Jack? What are you thinking
about?" I asked, and tried to ignore the mounting queasiness
of fear. There was a sadness, a depression, I'd never seen in
him before. But I saw it now. I saw it in his eyes. Not terror,

not self-pity, but the dull gnawing of insecurity, the deep
bruise of doubt.

"What are you thinking?" I asked. "Tell me."

"What if I don't get return?" Jack said in a monotone, still
staring at the ceiling. "They said two to three weeks. It's almost two. I haven't let it get me down. This is the first time
I've really been depressed."

"I don't know what you'll do . . . what we'll do if you
don't get return," I said. "I wouldn't have known what I'd
have done if someone had told me a year ago that you'd be
in an accident, in a hospital. I guess I wouldn't have believed
them."

"But if I'm paralyzed. If I can never walk. If we can never
make love."

I realized how contagious fear was, how, as a child, the
littlest hint of parental panic had terrified me, made me feel
lost and dizzy. I tried to fight the dizziness, the swirling feelings of doubt and questioning. I couldn't give in. *We* couldn't
give in. "Jack. I don't know what will happen. It will never
be the same. No, we've both changed, even though I can't
say how. But the most important is us. Not letting our personalities change. It's all now, all present. All I know is I love
you now, that I'm here, not because it's my duty, but because
I want to be here. Because I want us. I can't think about the
way we were. What's the point? You can't give in to the
ifs—if you hadn't taken that wave, if I hadn't wanted to go in
for that swim, if you don't get return."

"But we have changed," Jack said. "You said we've
changed. What do you mean, not let our personalities
change?"

I knew what I was thinking. I was fighting, fighting back
the fear. If Jack had doubts, they infected me. "I mean if
our life together became unbearable, unhappy, joyless, I
couldn't hide it from you. I *wouldn't* hide it from you. I

mean, we can't ever play games. We never have. I can't imagine being your nurse, living a life without sex. But we've had no sex for weeks, and if someone had told me two months ago that I wouldn't make love for two days, much less two weeks, I'd have told them they were crazy. Don't you see, Jack? Maybe one day I won't love you, but now I can't imagine that because I do love you. I don't see you as a cripple because you don't see yourself as a cripple. That's what I mean about personalities changing. Maybe we won't make it. Maybe one day I'll leave you or you'll want me to go, but that thought now makes me sick. If we change, we'll be two different people. And we'll know. But now I don't know those people. I can't even imagine them."

I felt flushed and excited. It was the fight that saved me from the dejection of hopelessness. It was the deep conviction that comes from loving someone that made me rebel against the odds. Jack was smiling at me and I smiled back. What a crazy time to feel lucky, to feel proud and strong.

Libbie and Lou had come into the room. They usually came in the afternoon, and their presence made me feel awkward. I could tell that Jack was disappointed they had picked that moment to visit. They knew they'd interrupted something, but they didn't know how to leave. There was something pathetic about the awkwardness, the need to play-act, to pretend that our roles ensured intimacy. For at this moment Libbie and Lou were strangers, and I felt like an actress who's forgotten her lines and waits helplessly for the prompter's whisper.

"And how's everything today?" Lou said in a mock-casual singsong. "And how's my little doll?"

"I'm okay," I heard myself say and watched Libbie caress Jack's face as she kissed him on the cheek. The room was hot and muggy.

"I brought you some fruit Jell-O," Libbie said. "I thought

something light might refresh you."

Jack thanked her, and some more small talk ensued. I knew they wanted to ask Jack if anything had happened, if there'd been the slightest movement, the tiniest sign of inward or outward improvement. Though they didn't ask out loud, their faces silently begged for some good news. I wanted to cry out, to ease the paralytic tension. At the same time that I wanted to draw them close to me, I wanted to confront the repressed feelings. And I also wanted to send them away. There was so much I wanted to tell Jack, now, right this minute.

"Is everything all right?" Libbie asked, sensing the tension.

"I'm just hot and uncomfortable," Jack said. "And we were talking. That's all."

"Well, we'll go," Libbie said. "We just stopped in to say hello."

"Don't be silly," I said, breaking the polite trance that seemed to hypnotize us all. "Why should you go? I'd like a break anyway. I didn't have a chance to buy the paper this morning. Stay awhile. I'll be back in a few minutes."

For the first time I felt trapped. I couldn't go back into that room. I couldn't go home. I wasn't hungry. I didn't really have to buy the paper; I'd already read it. I wished I could run away, away from families, away from problems. . . . No. I just wished the accident had never happened.

jack

I was so involved with myself that Mary was really the only person to whom I could talk. Mike and I kidded a lot and tentatively got to know each other, but we didn't really talk. And there just wasn't that much I could say to either Mary's or my family.

My parents would always ask me how I was coming along, and when I said nothing was happening, they tried to hide their disappointment. The questions annoyed me. It was a reminder that nothing had happened so far. I began shutting them out in self-defense. Mary and I were building our own world, always hoping for the best, but quietly preparing for the worst.

I knew how difficult it was for my parents. They had to adjust to the idea that Mary, someone they'd met only twice, was the person I needed most. She was the person whom I looked to to satisfy my needs; she controlled the traffic of visitors, dealt with the doctors and nurses, and with our close lawyer friend, Duff, took care of my outside affairs. She was the one in whom I confided. My parents were forced to trust and listen to the advice of a twenty-four-year-old woman simply because that was what I wanted.

I could tell they were confused. They'd flown across country to be with me, and when they arrived, they'd found there was not much they could do. Yet just having them there was good for me, though in actual fact I saw them very little. They would drop by the hospital at lunchtime with my favorite sandwich and would come by after dinner, usually with a malted or snack of some kind. It wasn't lack of imagination that kept them from doing more; it was that there was nothing else I wanted them to do. They were three thousand miles from home, in an unfamiliar place, only because of me. Yet they had to suffer the frustration of not even being able to be with me when they wanted because I needed Mary more.

Mary's parents were different. Obviously they felt awful about my personal tragedy. They had canceled their trip to Europe and had moved into our farmhouse to be with Mary and to help me. Norman had done everything he could to make sure I got the best care possible. Like my parents, they were with me almost every day. But there was the difference in attitude. My father was eternally, overwhelmingly confident, my mother had quiet hope (shored up completely by my father), and I felt Mary's parents were pessimistic, a pessimism born of a sense of reality and of real concern for her own best interest.

They had to be thinking about Mary's happiness first. I wasn't their son. I was the guy whom they hardly knew, who was engaged to be married to their daughter. And who now, according to the doctors, was almost certain to be paralyzed for the rest of his life. Who could blame them, I thought, if they thought how much better it would be if Mary and I split up. And that the sooner she saw this and started a new life of her own, the better. I felt they had to be thinking that. Hell, I was thinking it.

I thought about our breaking up, but I never reached any conclusions. I still hoped for return. If I didn't get it, then we would have to decide what to do. But until that time, there was an unspoken agreement between us not to discuss either our past, which would have been too painful, or our future, which seemed too ominous. I tried to examine my feelings. Did I feel guilty about the accident? No. Did I feel guilty about Mary? No. Was I dependent on her? Yes. Was I in any way encouraging her to stay by me by making her feel guilty or playing on her sympathies? No. So the hell with it, I thought. I was giving myself from two to four weeks to see if I would get any return. All my judgments and decisions were suspended while we waited out that time together.

One day when my parents and Mary were visiting with

me, a man came to the door of my room. He took a few steps and then hesitated. "Jack?"

For a moment I didn't know who he was. Then it hit me. "Stuart. My God, what are you doing here? How'd you know?" He tried to reply, but I didn't let him. "You remember my parents? And this is my fiancée, Mary Pleshette. Stuart and I were in school together. I can't believe it. I haven't seen you in thirteen or fourteen years," I said in wonder. "You look great. How'd you find me?"

By now he was all the way in the room and was smiling at my surprise. "I was in New York on a buying trip and called home to L.A. My wife, Barbara, told me what had happened. Someone had heard about the accident from your brother. I got on a train and here I am. I have to be back in L.A. tomorrow, so I can't stay long."

I couldn't believe he'd come all this way to see me. It was crazy but wonderful. I'd known him and his wife in school. He was a couple of years older than I, and we had never been particularly close. I rarely saw him after graduation, and I hadn't been in touch with him since I'd come to New York ten years before.

"Do you still see Freddy or Greenie?" I asked.

"We see a lot of Greenie. We've pretty much lost touch with Dave and Marilyn."

"I guess it's kind of a shock to see me like this after so many years. But we're just waiting to see what happens. The doctors still don't know for sure."

Stuart didn't say anything for a while. "Your spirits seem pretty good," he said. "You seem to be fine."

I asked him to sit down, but he insisted that he had to go. My parents offered to drive him to the station. They got up to go. "I'm glad I came," he said.

"Yeah. Me too," I said. "Say hello to everybody in L.A. for me." I couldn't get over it. He had come all this way after all this time to see me. I wondered what he knew about the accident, whether he really understood how bad things were. I also wondered what he and my folks were talking about on their way to the station and what he'd say about me to everybody in L.A.

One morning just before the two weeks were up, Joe went through his usual flexing, twisting, and bending of my limbs. "Try to move your toes," he said.

I tried. "I can't."

He told me to concentrate. "Think about your toes. You've somehow got to get the message down from your head through your central nervous system to your toes. Just try. Keep on trying."

I closed my eyes and concentrated as hard as I could on my toes. I felt nothing and nothing happened. It was as though my head were separated from my body. When I was a kid my father tried to teach me to wiggle my ears. I'd sit for hours, jiggling my scalp, crinkling my nose and forehead to no avail. But one day I felt something, and I realized I had to reach farther back for my ears. I stopped wiggling my scalp and concentrated on my ears. All of a sudden they wiggled. I now tried to concentrate on exactly the muscle I wanted to move. I tried to move my toes for a couple of minutes but still felt nothing. Finally Joe told me to relax and walked out of the room.

A few minutes later I tried to move my toes again. I tried to get a mental picture of the nerve circuitry, to picture the location of my toe. Suddenly I heard Mike hollering. "Your toe, your big toe is moving!" It was. I could feel the connection. I couldn't see it, but if I concentrated, I could will it to move. Mike called Joe back into the room, and I moved it for him. Then all the nurses crowded into the room for a look.

"What does it mean?" I asked Joe.

"I don't know," he said. "It could be the beginning of return or it could be nothing more than the fact that you can wiggle your toe."

"Come on. Commit yourself, damn it. I'm doing it. It's almost time. The two weeks are almost up. The swelling in my spine is going down."

"I don't know," Joe said, controlling the excitement I could hear in his voice. "You don't know. Don't kid yourself. Waiting is the name of the game. I can't predict what will happen. Just keep trying to move that toe. We'll see. We'll wait and see."

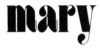
mary

"We've all been waiting for you," Janet LaVinio said with a big smile on her face.

I didn't know what she was talking about, but I rushed into Jack's room. I didn't have time to suspect or anticipate anything. Jack gave me a warm, glowing smile. "I have a surprise for you," he said, almost laughing.

"What? What's going on around here?" I asked.

"I can move my toe," Jack said. "I moved it late last night. . . ."

"What?" I said, not believing. "How? How did it happen? Tell me. Tell me everything."

"Joe asked me to try to concentrate on moving my toes. I tried. Shit. I broke my ass, but nothing happened. Then, just as he was out of the room, Mike started yelling. 'It's moving. Your toe is wiggling.' "

I listened, not believing. I was laughing at the ridiculousness, the hugeness, the sheer beauty of a wiggling toe. "Tell me again. Tell me everything that happened."

"I just told you." Jack was laughing too. "I called Joe back into the room and really concentrated, and he saw it move. I thought he was going to die. 'You did it,' he screamed. 'You wiggled your toe.' Mary, it's all so crazy. I can't see my feet, but I can tell when the toe moves. It's like I'm making a connection. I can't explain it."

I ran around to the foot of Jack's bed. His feet were propped up against a board. "Let me see. See if you can do it again."

"You have to move the board first," Jack said excitedly.

I stared at Jack's feet. I was concentrating so hard that my eyes hurt. I was scared to look at his face for fear of missing the sight of his toe moving. Nothing happened. And then it happened. The big toe on his left foot made a little bow and I could hear myself yelp with glee. "Oh, my God. It moved.

Oh, Jack. You really moved it. Do it again. Let me see it
again." I stared hard at his foot, hardly breathing, believing
that silence would somehow help him to do it again. I
watched that foot, the way a crowd at a circus watches a
tightrope walker, silently praying, immersed in excitement
and fear.

"I'm not moving it, am I?" Jack said, staring up at the
ceiling.

"No. It's not moving."

"There it goes," Jack said, his eyes wide with joy, his whole
face proud with accomplishment.

"You're right. Oh, Jack. You moved it again. I saw it. I really saw it. Tell me again what happened. Tell me what it all
means."

"Well, you know Joe," Jack said with a smirk. "He said it
might mean that I'm beginning to get return and that more
will follow. But it might just be that I can wiggle my toe and
that's it."

"He doesn't say more than that?" I asked.

"No."

Janet LaVinio had come into the room to give Jack his
little yellow pill. She was never mysterious about what was
going on. From the first day she'd told me what was happening with Jack. The morning after the operation she'd told
me that he was running a high fever, and when I looked
upset, she'd put her arm around me and said: "Mary, Jack
has just undergone major surgery and we have no idea how
much water he swallowed or how much sand was ground
into him when he was hurt. I can't tell you not to worry. But
he's fighting, his whole body is fighting. The fever is expected."

"Janet, what does it mean? Is it really something we can
get excited about?"

"I think it's worth getting excited about," she said. "Any

movement is good. It means that some signal is being sent through the cord."

I watched Janet drop the pill into Jack's mouth and slip the curved straw between his lips. She had white, smooth skin that always looked moist and cool. She wiped Jack's forehead with a washcloth and then rubbed his arms with her strong, clean hands.

I wanted to run home to tell everyone what had happened. "What can we tell your parents and mine?" I asked Jack.

"I guess all you can tell them is that I can move my big toe."

My mother was in the kitchen preparing lunch. I burst into the house like the kid who has no cavities in the Crest commercial. "Jack moved his toe. Papa? Did you hear? Jack can move his big toe."

They were happy but not jubilant. Their enthusiasm was guarded, and I felt the same kind of letdown one feels after telling a Great Joke which elicits only a polite chuckle instead of a belly laugh. "But it really is great news," I said to myself. "I just didn't tell it right."

I couldn't tell what it was in their eyes that disappointed me, made me sink with insecurity. I realized that I was a little girl again and that realization depressed me. I needed to please them. I needed the kind of affirmation I hadn't needed in years. I knew how fond they were of Jack, but that affection was measured by my happiness. I remembered with amusement my mother's reaction to my last boyfriend. She seemed to like him a great deal until we broke up. "I never liked that guy," she said. "I always had a feeling he was a neurotic no-goodnik." It was as though I were viewing the movement of that toe through the magnifying lens of a telescope where everything looked big and soft around the edges, while they were viewing it all through the long lens where the same objects looked razor-sharp and far away. To me, that toe took up the whole picture. To them, it was the tiniest, most distant dot in a frame so large that it almost didn't exist at all.

I didn't dare be hopeful. If I let myself think about how wonderful it would be if Jack's legs continued to come back and if he might walk again someday, I was overwhelmed by a terrible dread that some unseen force would punish me for even thinking those happy thoughts. Indulging in sanguine fantasy was a terrifying setup for disappointment. Wishing became synonymous with bad luck—"if I think about it or want it, it won't happen." I was vulnerable again. What if Jack's toe was some sadistic, horrible joke and was all that was coming back? I began to build up childish, superstitious conditions to ensure safety for my wishes.

As I left the hospital every night, I looked up at the sky and picked out the biggest and most glittering star. I would try not to blink, to keep my eyes glued to the flickering light for as long as it took me to make my wish. "Oh, please, let everything be okay. Let Jack walk again, let us be able to make love, let us be able to have babies, let him be able to use his hands." I'd try to make sure I wasn't forgetting anything. "Let his bowels and bladder return . . ." If people passed me and saw me mumbling to myself, straining my neck and staring transfixed at the sky, I didn't care. I wasn't even aware of them. After I finished my prayer, I felt tremendously relieved and not in the least bit silly.

jack

Every chance I got I tried to wiggle my toe. Sometimes it worked, sometimes it didn't. I was stretched out flat on the frame and couldn't raise my head to see my feet, but I knew it when I moved my toe. I'd test myself by checking with Mike or Mary. I could tell when I made a connection, no matter how weak. Somewhere inside my spinal cord there was a bruised nerve or ganglion that was healing, and if I concentrated I could locate it and send a message from my brain down through the cord into the muscle that controlled my toe. And even if the muscle was tired and my toe didn't move, I knew I was sending the message down that single live passage, because somehow I "felt" it.

The night I first moved my toe, my legs began doing a St. Vitus's dance, as if they were possessed. I would lie there, my legs outstretched, perfectly straight, and then one leg or the other would jump. Sometimes just a foot moved; other times my whole leg would bend at the knee. I'd try to stop it, but I couldn't. Then I'd try to take advantage of the involuntary motion to move my legs at will. But I couldn't do that either. The movement kept me up most of the night. It was as though I had developed a giant tic that didn't stop, that I couldn't control.

Joe didn't know what caused it, and he didn't know whether it really meant anything. It still excited me because, even if it was involuntary, at least I was moving. But days passed, and nothing else seemed to be returning. I had only sporadic control of my toe, and that was really hit-or-miss. The meagerness of the return began to get me down. Joe was right. I couldn't expect anything.

For a few days I thought I'd been getting feeling in my hands. One night I thought I could move them a little. I thought I could pinch my thumb and forefinger together. I showed Joe. He grabbed my wrist and held it tightly. Then

he told me to try to bend the forefinger. I couldn't. "Okay,"
I admitted. "I can't do it. I guess I was kidding myself, but I
do think I'm getting feeling back in my right hand."
Joe just laughed. "I think you're bulling me."
He was right. I had been kidding him and myself. There
was no more feeling in my hands. I began to get depressed
again. Mary, too, I could tell, was disappointed, but she
never said anything about it. She never asked if there was
any more return. She knew I'd tell her.
One afternoon I was lying on my stomach when my father
came barging into my room. He was full of enthusiasm because of the movement in my toe. I was depressed and feeling sorry for myself because there'd been no recent return.
He wanted to hear all about the return, but I just turned
him off by telling him that I was glad to see him but that it
was too hard for me to talk on my stomach. Anyway, I
wanted to sleep. I told him I'd see him that night.
When he and my mother came back to visit that night, I
was talking with Mary and her younger sister, Annie, who
had recently returned from Europe. My father prowled
around them like a trapped animal, impatient and angry. Finally I asked everyone but him to leave. He asked me how I
felt and immediately wanted to see me move my toe. His enthusiasm and optimism annoyed me. I knew it shouldn't, but
I couldn't help it.
"Look," I said angrily. "You can't get too excited. It's not
realistic. Just because I've got a couple of muscles doesn't
mean I'll get any more. I may never walk again, and you and
Mom have got to accept that. Calm down. You're not helping anybody. I may be in a chair the rest of my life. Don't
you understand that?"
He didn't say anything—he just looked at me. I could hear
myself, and I knew I sounded obnoxious. But I couldn't
stop. "You have got to be realistic, Dad. You can't expect im-

provements every day. You've got to expect the worst." I took a deep breath and waited. He outlasted me. "I'm sorry, Dad. Damn it. I'm down and it's been hot all day. It's not your fault."

He apologized for pacing the room and said it was just because he was so concerned about me. After he left, I lay there thinking about him and realized I'd never really explained anything to him, had never shown him how I could move. I'd shut him out.

He came back in the next day as if nothing had happened the night before. "Hiya, Jacko. How're you feeling?"

"Dad. I've been thinking about last night. Let me explain to you what I know. If the cord isn't torn, the reason I can't move is that it's badly bruised and swollen. That's putting pressure on the nerves. It may take up to four weeks for that swelling to go down. Understand?"

He nodded.

"But we don't know whether the cord was torn or how badly it was bruised. So we're just waiting. The toe coming back is a good sign, because it means that at least one nerve is intact. But it's possible that that's the only nerve or that there are just a few others. Nobody knows."

I realized I was lecturing, but I couldn't help it. He had to be made to understand. "Mary and I are hopeful, Dad. We really are. But we're afraid to get too hopeful because we've got to be prepared for the worst. We've got to live each day as it comes. I'd go crazy if I lay here and kept asking myself why there wasn't more return. And Mary would go crazy if she got up every day expecting something to happen and it didn't. I'm trying. I'm trying all the time to make connections. And I'm hopeful. And I'll tell you as soon as something does happen. In the meantime all we can do is keep our cool, and you've got to understand that."

He nodded, his blue eyes sparkling. I knew I was getting

through. Finally. He was pleased we were talking with each
other, dealing with it together. But I knew his way of dealing
with it was not to admit to himself that I might not make it.
Oh, he would handle it if I didn't get better. But he was in-
capable of anything less than pure optimism, and I knew he
was expectant each day. He needed that as much as Mary,
and I needed to take each day as it came.

A couple of days later Joe came into my room while I was
over on my stomach. He bent my right leg up from the knee
and then down again, taking me through the range of motion exercises he usually performed in the mornings. Then
he grasped my foot and swiveled the ankle, first to the right
and then to the left. "Okay, move your toe," he said.

I tried. I concentrated on the toe on my right foot, the one
that had never moved. Nothing happened.

"Relax," he said. "Try moving the left toe."

I tried and felt it move slightly.

"Good," he said, and then bent my left leg at the knee. As
he started to lower it, I tried to resist him. I thought I'd been
able to resist Clive a few times but was never sure. And I
could never do it for Joe. But this time I felt something. Joe
was pulling my leg down and I *was* resisting him, I was con-
sciously holding my leg up.

"Are you trying to do that?" he said.

I could only grunt "yes," I was concentrating so hard on
holding my leg back.

"Relax," Joe ordered, and set my leg down on the frame.
Then he bent it up again. "Okay, I'm going to pull the leg
down and you try to hold it back." He gripped my ankle
with one hand and placed his other hand behind my knee.
Slowly but steadily he began to pull my leg down toward the
frame.

I concentrated on my legs and held back with everything I
had. Slowly but steadily he was forcing my leg down, but I

was resisting him—I could feel it. And then Joe slapped my leg on the frame.

"I felt it," Joe cried. "I felt it. I could see it flex. You've got your hamstring. You've got it." He ran outside and called in the nurse. "Watch," he said and lifted my leg. I felt him slowly push my leg down toward the bed, and I held back.

"Look. Look," he cried. "The hamstring. It's quivering."

I resisted until I couldn't any longer and let my leg fall. I lay there staring down at the floor, totally exhausted. Joe was laughing, and I could hear the nurse laughing with him.

"You've got it. You've got your hamstring. I saw it quiver. It's only a quiver, but it's a beginning, Jack, it's a real beginning."

After Joe left, the nurses rolled me onto my back and turned out the lights. I tried sleeping but couldn't.

"Mike. You awake?"

"Yeah. I'm up."

"I can't sleep."

"Me either. Jesus. I thought Joe was going to buy champagne for the house."

"I can't believe it, Mike. I can't believe it. I've got that leg, it's okay. I just know it."

I lay awake for another hour and said to myself over and over, "I'm going to walk. I know I'm going to walk."

mary

"What did you say? You moved your leg? The whole leg?"
Jack was laughing as he described what had happened the
night before. "My hamstring. Joe screamed about how I was
resisting him. And then he said he could feel the muscle
behind my knee. He could feel it quiver." Jack looked like he
was going to cry. His lips trembled and his eyes filled with
tears. He never said the word "walk," but that's what we both
were thinking. This was more than a toe, the faint hint of
life; this was a whole leg, a real promise. I wanted to hear it
described again, just as I had when Jack first moved his toe.
Hearing it repeated was like rereading an especially marvelous chapter in a book. As Jack began to describe the excitement and discovery the previous night, it hit me.

"He's going to walk," I thought to myself. "I bet he's really
going to walk." And then I felt like weeping, as much from
my recurrent, superstitious fear that because I'd said it out
loud I had tempted fate, as from joy. I wrapped my arms
around Jack's body and kissed him. I pressed myself against
him, careful not to hit the tongs with my arms, nervous
about jerking his neck in my desire to be physically close to
him. I felt Jack awkwardly trying to caress my back and hair.
We were both laughing and crying.

"Can I feel the muscle?" I asked, walking down to the end
of Jack's bed. I pulled the sheet back and removed the board
which braced Jack's feet, almost black with the dead skin of
old sunburn. His right leg began to shake violently like a
machine gun when it's being fired.

"A spasm," Jack said, and waited for the jerky movement
to subside.

I slid my right arm underneath Jack's left leg and lifted it.
It felt heavy and sinewy as I awkwardly tried to hold the
back of his knee in my hand. I was shocked at how thin his
legs were, even though I had always teased Jack about hav-

ing thin legs before the accident.

"Grab my ankle with your left hand," Jack ordered. "That's it. Now I'm going to try to push down, but don't you move."

"Okay, I'm ready when you are," I said, and watched Jack's face strain and redden in effort. Then I felt a delicate flutter in his leg, as though the muscle beneath the smooth skin behind his knee had whispered to me. "I felt it! I felt it move!" I almost cried the words.

As I drove home for lunch, I realized I was happy, actually happy. I knew that our close friends, the Wardenburgs, were coming out to visit, and I couldn't wait to tell them the good news. Jack had known Fred for ten years and had made his first film with him. I also knew that despite my parents' quiet pessimism they, too, would be happy.

I saw Chris Wardenburg holding her baby, Jason, on her lap. She was sitting on the lawn talking with my mother. I ran over to them, bursting with excitement. "I have wonderful news," I said, bending over to kiss Chris and the baby. "Jack moved his leg last night. He can move his left leg."

My mother's face broke into a smile. "How wonderful," she said quietly.

Both Chris and Fred were anxious to see Jack, but I sensed they were also frightened. They had no idea what to expect and, like so many friends who had been in touch only by phone, were still stunned by the first horrible reports.

Jason wasn't allowed in the hospital, so Fred stayed with him while Chris and I went in to see Jack. I went in first to make sure Jack wasn't asleep. I beckoned to Chris to come in, and she hesitated at the door as though she wanted to turn and run. But Jack's face lit up with a huge grin when he saw her, and Chris seemed pulled to him like a magnet. She bent over and kissed him.

"You look great," Jack said, completely at ease, as though

he were lying on the beach or sitting in the Wardenburgs'
living room in Brooklyn.

"Oh, I'm so glad we finally got here," Chris said almost in
a whisper, a hospital whisper. I could tell she was upset by
the tongs and Jack's pallor, but also that she really was
happy to see him. I realized how strange the dark, claus-
trophobic room must have felt to Chris . . . to me? I always
rediscovered the inhumanity of the hospital through other
people's eyes.

Chris stayed only a short time. She said she'd wait outside
the front entrance of the hospital. I told her I'd join her
shortly.

"I know how badly Fred wants to see you, Jack," she said.
"I'll come back. But for now I think he should have some
time with you."

I watched Chris leave. I couldn't tell what she was feeling,
but I knew she was confused. She must have forgotten what
I had said about good news—the beginning of return—the
moment she saw Jack. She must have seen only human dev-
astation, for to the uninitiated eye Jack must have looked
devastated, physically destroyed.

I waited for Fred to come in before going out to join Chris
and the baby. I guessed she would want to be alone for a few
minutes. Fred was less timorous and clasped Jack's hand in
his. "I hear you moved a leg," Fred said. "That's great, really
great."

"Not really the leg," Jack said, "just the hamstring, but it's
a beginning."

"I'll leave you two alone for a while," I said, and went out
into the sunny day to sit with Chris and Jason.

"What's going to happen with Jack?" Chris asked.

"Seeing him really upset you, didn't it?" I said, trying to
sound understanding. I didn't want Chris to feel embarrassed or ashamed, and yet I was disappointed that Jack

obviously looked so bad to her.

"I guess it did. It took a lot out of me. I feel physically drained. What a joke that *I* feel tired! Oh, I hate myself for that."

"Don't hate yourself," I said, laughing. "What did you expect? I'm with Jack every day. I'm not aware of the change. I don't know what's going to happen. Neither of us does. Originally the doctors said he'd never walk again, but now I'm not so sure. To tell you the truth, Chris, we don't talk about what we're going to do . . . because we just don't know."

I knew that Chris understood what I was saying but that she couldn't really understand. I think people secretly expected to be saviors, or at least helpers, when they came out to visit us. I think the accident was so frightening and incomprehensible that it was a threat—the worst thing anyone could imagine; for some, worse than death. That it had happened to Jack, to a close friend, meant it couldn't be quickly or easily pushed out of mind. Somehow it had to be dealt with. But how?

The despondency many people felt after seeing Jack came simply from a lack of preparation to deal either emotionally or imaginatively with all the horrors Jack *was* dealing with. Every individual had his own secret dread, and I discovered that Jack became a weird human mirror to their deepest emotions and nightmares. It hadn't happened to them . . . yet. Ironically, the dread and threat of its happening to Jack was no longer. Strangely, he was freer than the rest. He had been reduced to the most basic honesty, to the purest openness . . . and many people weren't prepared for that. They came wanting to help, and left realizing that Jack had helped them, that in some strange way they had learned something new about themselves. They came expecting to listen, to be a shoulder to cry on, and left aware that they had done all the talking, all the confessing.

I went back to Jack's room. Fred and he were talking, and Mike was drunkenly raving in the background, high from his shot of Demerol. As I approached Fred and Jack, I noticed how big Fred looked. I'd known before the accident that they were about the same size, but now Fred seemed a giant. He was wearing a short-sleeved pullover, and I noticed how thick his forearms were. I had never thought I was particularly sexually attracted to him, but for a moment, seeing him standing next to Jack, I felt something stir and realized that I was reaching to the sight of a healthy man's body.

I felt embarrassed and frightened. I tried not to look at Fred in comparison to Jack. But I couldn't keep my eyes from darting back and forth between them. I saw Jack's thinness and pallor more clearly. I simply hadn't noticed the greasiness of his hair and the milky overcast of his eyes. For the first time I saw how much weight he'd lost (it was more than twenty-five pounds). It was as though his whole body had shrunk a size, like a sweater that is accidentally thrown into the washing machine and comes out familiar but totally misshapen. I would push the thoughts out of my head. I wasn't ready to deal with them. I wasn't even ready to acknowledge the repressed doubts and hidden fears. For the first time since the accident the outside world had squeezed its way into the limited but protected world of the hospital. For the first time I was seeing and judging Jack through the eyes of the past, and I was shocked by what I saw. Earlier that morning I had been elated by the movement of Jack's leg and had allowed myself the luxury of thinking about his walking. Now, compared to Fred, to normalcy, that movement seemed such a tiny thing.

jack

It was incredible. I was suddenly being treated like a prize race horse. Nurses kept coming into my room and massaging my legs. And I showed off for everyone.

Clive said he had to see for himself before he would believe what he had heard. He turned me over onto my stomach, held my leg, and told me to resist him while he bent it downward. He yelled and whooped and carried on just as Joe had the night before.

"Stop it," I said, on the verge of tears again. "You knew we'd do it."

He stopped laughing and turned to me with his big brown eyes. "You don't know what it means to us," he said. "We work so hard with you. We're always hoping you'll be okay, and then suddenly it happens. You just don't know what it means."

Fred and Chris Wardenburg visited the hospital the day after I got return in my hamstring, and Mary showed me off as though I were a child prodigy, made me wiggle my toe and had them hold my leg so they could feel the hamstring quiver.

"Gee, that's great," Fred kept saying. But I could tell he was confused by our enthusiasm. I felt he was more upset by what I couldn't move than excited by what I could move. Other friends on their first visits had the same kind of reaction. They hadn't seen me when I couldn't move anything, hadn't spent the three weeks with us in desperate wait. They only saw me as I was—head shaved, tongs in my skull, immobile. They couldn't imagine where I'd been or what an achievement that toe and hamstring were, or what it meant to us.

Later that same day I felt as though I had to urinate but couldn't. Mary checked and saw that the catheter wasn't draining and called the nurse to fix it. That was the first time

I'd felt my bladder. Mary and I looked at each other but said nothing, afraid to get too excited about it, afraid the feeling had no real significance. But there were other signs. Every two days they gave me suppositories to try to regulate my bowel movements. The suppository was supposed to act within forty-five minutes. The first time they gave me one, nothing happened after forty-five minutes, so the nurse removed the bedpan. Four hours later, while I was on my stomach, I defecated. I had a childish sense of naughtiness and freedom lying there on my stomach and shitting.

The second time they gave me a suppository, I again messed the bed. I had absolutely no control over my bowels and felt no warning. I got depressed and scared. The next time, nothing happened after forty-five minutes, so I told the nurse to remove the bedpan. They began to wheel me out of my room on the way to X-ray, when I felt it coming. I told Clive to get the bedpan. He lifted me up and got it under me just in time. I'd felt it coming. More than that, I thought I was using my sphincter muscles to try to hold it back. I didn't know if those muscles had been there all along or if I'd used them for the first time.

I told Mary's father what had happened. "But I'm not really sure, Norman, if I did feel my sphincter muscle."

"If you think you feel a muscle, then you feel it," he said. I believed him.

The next day Joe tried my leg again and said it was a little stronger. I could resist him a little more. He grabbed my ankle and told me to move my foot. I tried to swivel it at the ankle, but I wasn't making a connection. It wasn't moving. I tried thinking about my knee. I tried to think about turning *it*. I tried "right" and then "left," but I wasn't making any connection there either. Then I thought about my heel, and I tried moving *it*. Again, I felt nothing, but Joe said, "You moved it. I think you moved it. Try again." So I thought about my heel again and tried to remember what I had just done. "You did it," he said. "You did it again. I saw it move. Try again." I tried, but nothing more happened. "Put my leg down, Joe. I'm tired." He put it down and picked up the other foot. But I couldn't make it move so he tried the left one again. "Okay, move your heel," he said. I concentrated on my ankle and heel. "You did it again," he said excitedly. "That muscle is an extension of your hamstring. It all figures. You've got three down and only nine hundred muscles to go."

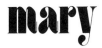
mary

After Fred's and Chris's visit with Jack, we went back to the house and talked.

"Do you have any idea what's going to happen?" Fred said. "What have the doctors said about sex? Do they think Jack'll be able to screw?"

I was shocked by his directness but tried to hide my feelings. "They say we'll be able to," I said. "But they don't know about children. . . . It's still too early to know anything definitely."

I felt Fred was freer to question me than he was Jack, and I couldn't completely blame him for his curiosity. Sex was probably the first thing everyone wondered about. The question he posed with uninhibited candor presumed a separation or distance between Jack and me, as though I were an objective bystander who could comment coolly on the fate of his friend. But I wasn't an outsider. I was part of that fate, part of the answer to these questions. "Will he be able to screw?" meant will I be able to screw. What would happen to Jack was what would happen to me. To the outside world I was a free agent, a young woman capable of forming new relationships. But to me freedom without Jack meant nothing.

I tried not to be angry with Fred, who, I knew, was asking these questions out of love and concern. Anyway, I reacted more violently to people who did a bad job of suppressing the same questions, like the mother of a friend who asked whether we were still planning on getting married. "What do you mean?" I said.

"Well—" she stuttered. "It's such a big decision."

"We're not rushing into it, if that's what you mean."

At least Fred came right out with it, like a child greedy for knowledge and understanding. But I realized I was more sensitive to the questions about sex than I had been earlier. Much more sensitive.

Shortly after the Wardenburgs' visit I got a phone call from a researcher at *Newsweek*. At first her voice, heavy with sadness, was unrecognizable and seemed to be directed at someone else. The people who'd just learned of the accident always sounded peculiar to me, for as time passed, the consuming pressure of crisis had begun to dissipate and I felt progressively calmer and more in control.

"Things are really much better," I said, trying to comfort her. That's what was so strange about those phone calls. It was I who did the comforting, convincing them that everything was going to be all right.

"Well, when did it happen?" she asked. "I was away on vacation and sort of just heard. It sounded really bad, just *horrible*."

"Well, it's much better now," I repeated, not wanting to go into all the details.

There was a silence, and then she blurted out: "Christ, you sure must be horny." I couldn't believe what I was hearing.

"Libido's the first thing to go in a crisis," I said weakly, and told her I had to go. I couldn't move from my seat when I'd hung up the phone. The words, "You sure must be horny," kept running through my head. Why did she say that? Was I crazy, or was that the dumbest thing in the world anyone could say? I almost started to laugh.

I began to think of all the bright, nasty things I should have said in retaliation and then thought to hell with it. She hadn't meant to hurt me. And what was it that was really upsetting me? It wasn't just the crudeness of the question or the insensitivity of the thought. I felt that my innermost privacy was being invaded, that my lack of sex life had somehow become a matter of public concern. I realized I cared what other people thought, how they viewed a situation they knew virtually nothing about. I had never thought about what other people thought right after the accident. I hadn't had time. Now I hated the idea of people viewing me as a victim, a frustrated, unfulfilled victim. I imagined women at work and the mothers of friends sitting at Schrafft's wondering out loud, "Well, how can she marry him now? It would be tragic for a young girl like Mary to be saddled with a . . . a . . . cripple. I don't think paralyzed people can do it, do you?"

I told Jack about the phone call and how it had upset me. I described my sudden sensitivity to what other people said or thought about us.

"Maybe you're upset about what they're saying and thinking because that's what you're thinking but can't say," Jack said. "You have to be questioning and doubting all the things they are. I know I am. Sex has been such an important part of our life."

"And it will have to continue to be," I said. "But it will be different." I realized I needed Jack as much as he did me. The bond between us had strengthened, and the early carefree sexual intimacy had been replaced by an inexhaustible devotion. We knew we were no longer carefree, that we had lost a certain playfulness, but that's all we knew. Neither of us was ready to settle for anything less than normalcy at this point—although who knew what normalcy was. We shared a special intimacy which in its greatest intensity was sex. And mixed with our fear was hope.

jack

Though I never mentioned it to Mary, I was worried about the catheter. Did it mean I would never have control over my bladder? Could it do permanent damage? And most important, how had the accident affected my reproductive organs?

After the operation I'd asked Joe if I could fuck and he had said, yes, but that I probably wouldn't feel anything. I'd been too scared to consider the possibility of impotence or not being able to ejaculate. So like everything else that had to do with the accident, I tried to put it out of my mind and waited to see what would happen. But I couldn't totally block it out.

And now that it looked as if my leg was coming back, what worried me most was sex. I could imagine a relationship where we couldn't have children. It would be disappointing, but we could always adopt kids. But I couldn't imagine a relationship without sex. It was so much a part of us. The only "information" I had was that a few times I'd felt the catheter being inserted into my penis, although it had never been really painful. That I felt something gave me hope, but I didn't dare hope for too much.

Joe asked a urologist, a Dr. Weir, to examine me. The night he was expected I was tense. I wanted to know everything, but I was also afraid the news would be bad.

Dr. Weir came into my room pushing a rack with a half-dozen bottles suspended from it. The first thing he did was push his finger hard up into my scrotum. Normally I would have jumped, but of course I couldn't move and was too nervous and surprised even to complain.

"Does that hurt?" he asked.

"Hell, yes, it hurts."

Then he stuck my scrotum with a pin. I felt that, too. I was quietly thankful for the pain. Then he stuck me around my thighs and belly. It all felt dull. I could feel the pressure

of the pin sticking me but felt no pain. Why did I have feeling in my balls but not my thighs? I didn't understand, but I
knew somehow something was partially good.

Phyllis, the evening nurse, was standing by. I wished she
would leave. I didn't want her around when I asked Weir
questions. But he didn't give me much time to think about it.
He reached under me and shoved a finger up my rectum
and pressed my prostate. At the same time, he held my
penis. He squeezed the prostate. It hurt. He said my penis
had reacted. "That's very important," he said. "That's good.
It means you can have erections."

I smiled and sneaked a look at Phyllis, who was also smiling. "How come?" I asked. "How do you know?"

"The long nerves that run down into the penis and the
prostate are intact," he said.

That's probably why I can move one leg, I thought. But
does that mean if I can't move the other leg, there are
nerves that have been severed?

"How come I have sensation in my penis and scrotum but
not over the rest of my body?" I asked.

"I don't know," he said. "We really don't know much
about spinal injuries."

How strange, how lucky, I thought.

"Each case is different," he interrupted my thoughts. "You
know I was once paraplegic."

"You were?"

"I caught a bullet in the spine in Korea."

"But you're fine. You can walk beautifully."

"I've still got a brace on my leg, and I limp a little."

I hadn't noticed the limp. I still couldn't detect it. I didn't
know what kind of brace he had or even what it did. He was
up and about, apparently normal. He was walking.

It was good to know he'd been hurt like me. I knew he understood. But it was also the first time I'd thought of myself

as a paraplegic. In fact, I wasn't a paraplegic; I was a quadriplegic. The sudden realization, the connection of word to fact, shocked me. I thought of the World War II film *The Men* with Marlon Brando. I saw shattered skinny bodies in wheelchairs. I saw active, athletic, independent men turned into burdens to their families. I saw them being pushed around, waited on, bitter and angry. Paraplegic. The word numbed me. I suddenly saw myself as I really was. I attached an image to my accident, an image learned from movies. I vaguely wondered why I hadn't thought of myself as a paraplegic-quadriplegic before. I also wondered why I never heard the word around the hospital. Had Mary used it?

But maybe I didn't have to be a basket case. My left leg was coming back, and Weir said I could have erections. He said the signs in my genital area were good. I pressed him about paraplegics. I told him I thought I had a leg back, and now if I could get my cock in action (I didn't care that Phyllis was there) I'd be happy. Weir laughed. He told me he had a couple of spinal-injury patients. "One of them's a paraplegic," he said. "He's still in a wheelchair, but he's back at work. He can drive a car and gets around pretty well by himself. His sex life is lousy. But I think his problems are as much psychological as physical because I think he's capable of normal sex."

"What about the other guy?"

"He was a quadriplegic like you. He can walk now and has a normal sex life."

"You say I will be able to have erections, but will I be able to ejaculate?"

"It's too early to tell," he said. "And that's much more complex."

"When will I know?"

"You'll have to wait."

If I didn't have the catheter, I thought, I could try to masturbate. Finally Weir ran some tests on my bladder. He pumped fluid into it, measured the amount I could hold, and then, with both hands, pressed down on my bladder as if he were deflating an inner tube and pushed all the liquid out. It hurt.

"You may have to urinate by pressing on your bladder, just like that," he said. I heard him but wasn't listening. I was trying to absorb what I'd just learned about my sex life. The nerves were there. I had sensation, and that was important. I could get erections, and that was important. But maybe I couldn't ejaculate. What would sex be like without ejaculation? Don't think about it, I said to myself.

Weir pumped some more fluid into my bladder. "Is the water warm or cold?" he asked.

I couldn't really tell, but I thought it felt a little warm. "Warm," I said, unsure of myself.

"That's right. Good."

"I really couldn't tell," I confessed. "But I think it was warm."

"It doesn't matter," he said. "You were right."

mary

I knew Jack was going to see a urologist, and I was simultaneously anxious for him to have and not to have the prescribed tests. Not knowing was less and less of a comfort as time went on, but the possibility of knowing definitively that our sex life might be finished was unbearable. "Sex isn't everything," I remembered Joe saying. "Maybe not to you," had been my silent response. Of course sex wasn't everything. But what did that mean?

Luckily I didn't know which day Dr. Weir was coming. Unaware, I walked into Jack's room one morning and saw an extra bottle attached to his bed with a cord leading ominously in the direction of his crotch. Oh, my God, I thought to myself. This is it. It's worse than I imagined.

"The urologist was here late last night," Jack said.

"Well, what happened?" I almost shouted.

"Calm down. I'm telling you. He said he was very hopeful that I'd be able to have erections. He did all these tests, one where he stuck a pin in my balls."

"And you felt it?"

"Fuckin' A I felt it! He said the long nerves to my scrotum, bowels, and penis are intact. . . . But it's still too early to know about ejaculation. That's much more complicated."

I felt myself flush and weaken at the knees. I sat down and took a deep breath, not sure of my reaction to what Jack was telling me. It was neither as bad as I had dreaded nor as good as I had hoped. I wanted it all—erection, ejaculation, perfection. I wanted to be totally reassured that sex would be just as it had been. This was the one area where my tolerance for the unknown was abysmally low and where my expectations were dangerously high.

"What do you mean, he doesn't know about ejaculation?" I tried to be calm but knew I sounded accusatory.

"Just what I said. The whole mechanism for ejaculating is

very complicated, and there's no way he can test those nerves."

"I see. Tell me what he did."

I listened intently as Jack described the series of water tests, pin tests, pressure tests, and temperature tests the doctor had performed. The fuller the description, especially of what Jack was *feeling*, the more hopeful I became.

"So the pins really hurt you," I said. "You really felt them."

Jack and I laughed at my glee that he'd felt pain, genital pain.

"What did he say about the catheter? Will they take that out soon? Is it hurting you to leave it in?"

I knew I was being too insistent and perhaps asking too many questions, but I couldn't help it. Jack seemed to understand my compulsive need to be reassured. I hated my obsession, my minimally disguised panic. I'd lived through a month not knowing whether Jack would ever move a muscle again. I'd watched the slow and torturous return of his left leg and waited patiently for the progressive stirrings in his right. A month before I'd been able to imagine living with a man in a wheelchair. My idealized picture of us surrounded by children had even been a comfort. But now that picture frightened me.

As I walked out of the hospital toward the parking lot, I saw Joe slamming the door of his car.

"Jack tells me that Weir's report pleased you," I said.

"Yes, it did."

I waited to see if he'd say more—I hoped something reassuring.

"You know, Mary, your feelings about Jack might change. . . . You can't be too hard on yourself if they do. Jack is going to be a big responsibility, and you're very young."

"Don't all relationships change?" I said, feeling the bile

rise in my throat. "And don't you think that Jack and I know this?" I resented Joe's de-personalizing Jack by thinking of him more as a big responsibility than as a man.

"I'm just telling you this for you," Joe said. "Very few people really know what it's like."

"We don't pretend to know," I said. "So there seems no point in worrying now about how I'll feel two months or a year from now. Who would have thought Jack would have come this far three weeks ago?"

"You're right about that," Joe said. "But remember, I was the one who had hope."

"I haven't forgotten," I said. "So why lose it now?"

Joe bit on his pipe and forced a smile. He turned and walked up the steps toward the hospital.

I wasn't sure that he'd really heard what I'd just said.

And I really didn't care.

jack

One day while Mary and Norman were visiting with me, Joe came in. "You need another operation to stabilize your neck," he said. "We'll take some spongy bone from your hip and fuse it to the vertebra that's been damaged in your neck."

"When?" I asked.

"In about ten days. Afterwards I hope we will be able to move you within five or six weeks to a rehabilitation center, depending on how quickly you recover."

The idea of another operation didn't bother me. "It doesn't sound as dangerous as the first operation," I said. "You won't be working so close to the spinal cord."

Joe looked at Norman and then at me. "All operations are dangerous. There's the usual risk of disease and the dangers of anesthesia. But I'll have the top specialists in the field working with me, and we'll cut the risk as much as possible." Joe paused. "But I really have to tell you there have been a number of deaths from this type of operation due to unknown causes."

"What do you mean?" I said. "People you've operated on? How many? What caused it?"

"We don't know what caused it," he repeated. "I've never had it happen to one of my patients. I've just read about it in the medical literature."

I looked at Mary, who was watching me carefully. Norman was looking at Joe but didn't say anything. As he turned to leave the room, Joe said, "Don't worry. We'll take care of you."

That's just great, I thought.

"Are you scared?" Mary said.

"Hell, yes, I'm scared." What I didn't say to her was that I was afraid of dying. I'd never thought of dying before the first operation. I wouldn't have thought of it now if Joe hadn't mentioned it. I didn't question the risks in any operation. I figured the doctors knew what they were doing, that the operation was mechanical and by itself not dangerous, and that they were pretty sophisticated in handling postoperative complications. Why did Joe go out of his way to frighten me?

I couldn't sleep. I lay there panicked. I thought about the operation and about death—death from unknown causes. Something doctors had no control over. I was getting angry. He might as well have said, "Don't worry, there's nothing you can do. Thousands of people die in automobile accidents every year."

What the hell did that have to do with me? So the odds were in my favor. They were in my favor when I took the wave. After all, how many people break their necks bodysurfing?

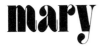

How they would take a tiny piece of bone from Jack's hip and fit it carefully into his cervical spine like a pivotal piece in a jigsaw puzzle fascinated me. I knew all operations were risky, but I was almost smug that this one would be okay.

"There have been a number of deaths from this type of operation due to unknown causes," Joe told Jack as my father and I stood around his bed. I watched Jack's eyes and then looked at Papa, who remained silent. No one said anything for quite some time, but I could feel that my father and I were holding back our anger, our desire to tell Joe what a stupid ass he was to mention death right before Jack was to be operated on. It was at moments like this that the doctor-patient relationship was nothing more than a source of frustration, and I resented Joe as a doctor even though I didn't really dislike him as a person. In fact, I rather liked him when he wasn't trying so hard to be a doctor. The only reason I didn't turn around and tell him he was a fool for frightening Jack was some misplaced, almost pathological respect for his position as doctor.

The flat voice of the head nurse came over the loudspeaker: "Visiting hours are now over. All visitors must leave by nine o'clock."

I grabbed Jack's hand and brought it to my lips. I didn't want to leave. I felt helpless to soothe his fear, and seeing it in his eyes made me frightened. "It'll be all right, Jack."

"I know it will, baby. Don't worry. I'll be okay. Give me a kiss and go home and get some rest."

Papa and I walked toward the car. "What do you think about Joe's saying that business about death from unknown causes?" I said.

"He was a dope to say that," my father said in his scratchy, gruff voice. "But he's young and insecure, especially around me. We all know that any time you take a general anesthetic you're risking death, but what's the point of saying it? This operation isn't nearly as dangerous as the first. They won't be working on top of the spinal cord, and Jack's in better shape going into the operation than he was the first time. And technically we know Joe's extremely capable."

"So you're not too worried?" I said, needing to be reassured.

"No," my father said. "It's amazing he's come this far. As long as he keeps improving . . ."

I didn't ask Papa what if he doesn't improve? I didn't want to know what he thought about that.

As soon as we got home, my younger sister, Annie, bounded toward me. "How about a game of spit before supper?" she said.

"Sure. But you'll have to teach me how to play again." I was glad she'd come home from Europe to be with us.

We sat down on the living-room floor and began to play. After a few games we were laughing hysterically, bending and throwing the cards in our race to win. "You cheated!" she screamed.

"No, I didn't."

"Oh, I'm tired anyway," she said, gathering the cards up.

"Just two more games," I said, disappointed that she'd had enough. It felt so good to be silly and childish. Sitting there on the floor, I felt free of all responsibility. I didn't have to think. And Annie always beat me anyway.

The alarm went off at six thirty, startling me out of a deep sleep. I could tell that it was going to be a hot day from the fuzziness of the horizon and the heaviness in the air. I didn't linger in bed any more because Jack wasn't there to linger with. And on this morning I wanted to get to the hospital by seven—a full hour before Jack would be wheeled into the operating room.

As I walked into the hospital I was struck by the amount

of movement and noise at such an early hour. If I'd been dropped inside those walls with no knowledge of the time of day, I certainly wouldn't have been able to tell whether it were morning, noon, or night. Like a wind-up clock the hospital seemed to run on its own time.

I could tell that Jack had been waiting for me to arrive. He looked tired but alert with anxiety. I could see in his eyes that he was scared. The pupils seemed fixed, as though they might not react to light—the whole eye staring but not seeing. I kissed Jack and felt the dryness of his lips.

"Don't you want something to drink?" I said, forgetting that you couldn't eat or drink before an operation.

Jack looked at me a little angrily. "Yeah, get me a tall gin and tonic—you know they won't let me," he said.

"You're scared, aren't you?" I said.

"Yeah. I've been awake half the night. It's crazy. Last time everyone was scared, and I didn't know it. Now they're all running around like they do every morning—same jokes, same everything, and I'm shitting in my pants."

I held Jack's hand in mine. It felt cold. "It's crazy," I said. "Because I think it's going to be okay, too. I know that's no help, but . . ."

"Yes, it is," Jack said. He looked at me and tried to smile a dry, crack-lipped smile.

A nurse came into the room holding a hypodermic needle in her hand. She hastily pulled the sheet off Jack's right leg and jammed the needle into his thigh.

"I felt that," he said excitedly. "That's the first time I've felt anything in my right thigh."

"That's where I plugged you," the nurse said gaily. "Right in the old thigh. That's great, Jack. You come out of that operation feeling a lot, too. Okay?"

"What did you give me?" Jack said before she left.

"Just something to relax you. A little morphine."

Two nurses dressed in green came into the room. "We're all waiting for you," one of them said, beginning to wheel the bed out of the room. "This is the first time the morphine hasn't worked," he said. "I guess I'm really scared." "It's going to be okay," I said, walking alongside the moving bed. "I'll see you later. I'll be here when you wake up, when it's over."

"I love you, Mary . . . I'll be okay."

I watched the bed move into the operating room—a frightening, forbidding place to me. I stood dumbly for a while, the way you stand after someone you love boards a plane and you've watched the last traces of exhaust disappear in the sky after take-off. I snapped out of my daze and repeated the words, "It's going to be okay," and left the hospital.

When I reached the parking lot, Libbie was just getting out of her car.

"They just wheeled him into the operating room," I said.

"Oh, no," she cried. "I didn't think the operation was till eight thirty or nine."

I could see how disappointed she was. I couldn't see her eyes behind the dark glasses, but I knew they were filling with tears. I felt incredibly sad for her.

"I know," I said, wrapping my arm around her waist. "Let's go inside and get some coffee."

Libbie hooked her arm around me and drew herself close as we walked back toward the hospital. Neither of us said anything, and for the first time in a long while I felt comfortable with the silence we shared. When I'd first seen her in the parking lot, I had felt a twinge of jealous resentment that she had come at all. I thought she should have known how important it had been for me to be alone with Jack. But now I realized how wrong I was to resent her. I remembered

what my mother had often said to me: "You'll never understand the pain a mother feels when her child is hurt or
disappointed until you have your own children. . . ."
Libbie had been so controlled and considerate all this time
that I felt ashamed that my tendency was to condemn her
self-control instead of appreciating her consideration. As my
mother had said, I couldn't really know the pain she was
feeling, but for the first time since the day she arrived, I felt
close to her, felt the love we both felt for Jack.

"George Wallach took this picture of Jack when he was
three and a half years old," Libbie said over coffee. She was
fondling a tattered photograph of a little boy with red hair
and masses of freckles splashed across his cheeks and nose.
He was smiling, his head cocked to one side, his big blue
eyes overflowing with warmth and sympathy.

"He really looks like an advertisement for Borden's Milk—
the wholesome American boy," I said. I realized I was smiling back at the photograph.

"We were still in Milwaukee then . . . I must have been
pregnant with Dick." Libbie sipped her coffee and seemed to
relax with her memories. I asked her to tell me more.

"Oh, Jack was a great little boy," she said. "He could be a
devil, but we all had such fun."

"How old was he when you moved to California?"

"Jack was nine and Dick was five. Jack always had a mind
of his own. He got sick a lot when he was young—lots of
colds, and pneumonia four times. But if he was feeling good
and I tried to keep him indoors, he'd always find a way to
get out and play baseball. Once he and Dick decided to prac-
tice their sliding outside the house. I remember because I'd
just cleaned up. By the end of the afternoon half the dirt
from the yard was inside the house."

She pulled some more snapshots out of her wallet—one of

Jack and Dick on the beach, both of them all teeth and spindly legs; their senior prom formal pictures; the one of Jack in a white dinner jacket and black bow tie, his hair cut short, his teeth white and even, his smile a little "1950s sincere." I figured that when that particular photo was taken, I was six years old, and I started to laugh.

"You know. I never think of the age difference between us," I said. "But do you realize that when Jack was graduating from Fairfax High, I was in first grade?"

Libbie and I both laughed. All that time behind us. It was easy to remember the good times. "Jack didn't know I existed when that picture was taken, and I'd never even heard of California." I realized I was thinking out loud. "I remember all those nights with girl friends, wondering who we'd marry, really wondering, knowing he existed somewhere, but not knowing who or where. It's all pretty crazy, isn't it?"

"I guess it is," Libbie said, lighting a cigarette. And I realized we were serious again, that we were sad.

"I think we should both go home and get some rest," I said. "I'll see you in a couple of hours."

jack

The afternoon before the operation they shaved my pubic hair, part of my head, and all of my chest, down to my navel. I was reminded of the hairless male models on the covers of homosexual magazines, but now with my very white skin and skinny body I felt more like a plucked chicken.

Ann, a nurse's aide, came into the room to say hello. "Let me see what you look like, honey," she said as she slid the sheet slowly and sensuously down my body.

"Hey, me too, baby," Mike yelled.

"You get yours later, honey," she promised.

Joe had agreed to let Mary be with me right up to the time of the operation. He also agreed to give me morphine instead of Demerol after I reminded him of my previous bad trip. "There's not much to be afraid of," was his parting shot.

Schmuck, not much for you to be afraid of, I thought.

Time dragged. I got more nervous. I developed a pain in my right side and was sure it was an appendicitis. The nurses came to give me an enema, but when I complained about the pain, they decided to call Joe. They didn't reach him until after ten that night. He came over to the hospital and examined me. He said, "It's just gas, forget the enema, go to sleep, and I'll see you in the morning."

I fell asleep and dreamed I was going to be operated on, but first I had to get over a twenty-five-foot wire playground fence. I started to climb over it. When I got to the top and looked down, I froze with fear, unable to move. I just clung to that fence, afraid to go forward or backward. I awoke thinking about the dream and death from "unknown causes." Finally I fell asleep again. When I awoke, Mrs. Swanson—Swanee—was there. "What time is it?" I asked.

"Around two in the morning."

"Can I have some water?"

"Sorry, chief. Nothing to eat or drink until after the

operation." She told me that a part-time substitute nurse named Martha, whom Mike and I had dubbed "super-sub," had called to wish me luck and to tell me that she would be in Thursday night to take care of me. Then Swanee bent down and gave me a big kiss on the forehead, "Good luck, chief."

I awoke too early—about six o'clock—and lay there thinking nervously about the operation until Mary came in about seven. Then a nurse came in to give me a shot.

"What's that for?" I asked.

"To dry out your mouth for the operation."

"To dry out my mouth! If it were any drier, I couldn't talk at all."

Then they wheeled me out of my room and down to the operating room. Mary walked beside me and kissed me before they pushed me through the big swinging doors into the operating area.

"See you, baby," I said, and we kissed again.

Joe came by and introduced me to Dr. Farrell, who was going to assist him in the operation. Then they went off to have coffee and study my X-rays. A nurse with a check list asked if I had any false teeth or allergies. An aide with a clipboard asked me the same questions. I felt like I was in a Marx Brothers movie. It struck me also that I didn't remember their asking me questions before the first operation, although they must have.

The longer I waited, the more nervous I got. I hated just lying there like a lump, while people were walking by me. I wondered what they thought when they saw me there. Did they think I might die? Did they try to imagine the pain I might feel?

Once I was actually wheeled into the operating room, I felt better. I was now not only part of the scene; I was the centerpiece. Now I could participate, even if my participation was only cooperative. An intravenous tube was stuck in my arm.

"Okay. Now we're going to feed you some oxygen." A rubber mask was put over my mouth and nose. I closed my eyes and took deep breaths.

"Now we're going to feed you the gas . . . just take a couple of deep breaths."

While I was wondering if I would be aware of going to sleep, I went under.

From a distance I thought I heard Joe talking to me. I tried to push through to him. Clearly I heard him say, "The operation was successful." I think I smiled, and then he said something about my legs which, if I heard, I didn't remember when I finally did come out of the anesthesia and was fully conscious in the Intensive Care unit. But by that time Joe was gone.

I hurt a little. One of the nurses gave me an injection and I felt better, even a little euphoric. The operation was over and I'd come through it successfully. I was almost smug. No thoughts now about death from unknown causes.

Janet LaVinio came in smiling. "I know this is against the rules and I'll probably get killed for it, but I had to come by and say hello."

Her smile was like a sunburst, and her eyes were twinkling. She showed me a pretty little lace hanky. "I carried this when I got married," she said. "I brought it today for good luck for you. I told Mary I wanted her to carry it when you two get married."

mary

"Jack wants you to know that he can still wiggle his toes," a kindly, round-faced nurse told me.

"When will I be able to see him?" I asked.

"He's still pretty groggy. Give him a couple more hours. We'll move him back to his room by then."

I was excited. The operation was over and Jack was alive, wiggling his toes. I saw Joe and ran up to him. He was still wearing his white operating shoes and gown. He was glowing.

"It went beautifully, Mary. He lost very little blood, and Dr. Farrell is very optimistic."

At that moment I felt nothing but love for Joe, and instinctively kissed him on the cheek. He was surprised and pleased. He led me over to a taller man who was also wearing a surgical gown. Dr. Farrell looked older than Joe, and his manner was friendly and relaxed. I held out my hand and he shook it warmly.

"I think Jack's going to make it," he said. "I think he's going to walk. I'm not as sure about his hands—but there's still a good chance they'll come back too."

I felt elated, mesmerized by his positive prognosis. I grabbed his hand. "Thank you so much," I said. "I can't tell you how much I appreciate your help."

Farrell smiled at me. "You don't have to thank me," he said. "Jack's an extraordinary guy. . . . Joe's told me how well you both have been handling this. . . . It's you who should be thanked."

Jack was still half asleep when they wheeled him back into the room. He had a small bandage on the front side of his neck. I found out later that the incision was only two inches long and ran along a natural crease line in his neck. When it healed, the scar would be no more than a large wrinkle in his skin, a vague reminder of hard times.

Jack moaned and tried to move his hand toward his right

hip. I gently lifted the sheet and saw a large gauze bandage
stuck to his side with adhesive tape. There was some blood
on the bandage, but it looked more like red paint than like
real blood. I couldn't understand what he was saying. I bent
forward to kiss his forehead and to hear him more clearly.
"My throat," he whispered. "My throat is killing me."
"Don't talk," I said. "You'll be fine. Just rest. The operation was a success. You'll be okay."
I offered him a glass of cold water. The straw slipped out
of his mouth as he weakly sipped it. As he swallowed, his
face tightened with pain, and I remembered my own first
excruciating taste of water after my tonsils had been removed ten years before.
I watched Jack fall back to sleep. Mike, too, was sleeping,
his mouth open and his head precariously balanced on the
edge of his pillow. It was getting dark. The whole day had
passed, and I felt strangely removed from time. The early-
morning drive to the hospital, the operation, the talk with
Libbie could have happened months before. I wasn't even
sure what day of the week it was.
As evening wore into night, Jack's discomfort increased. I
stayed by his side as much for my peace of mind as for his
comfort. At eight a group of Mike's friends barged into the
room. I'd seen them all before. They were always loud,
bragging about all the booze they'd drunk, grass they'd
smoked, and chicks they'd balled. It hadn't bothered me
before—in fact, they'd been something of a diversion. But
this night they really got to me; they seemed especially noisy.
A small, wiry guy who looked like a spider monkey lurched
into Jack's bed. A wave of hatred swept over me, and I
wanted to yell but could only stare coldly at him. He apologized meekly. Jack couldn't have felt the bump, but the
monkey didn't know that. I drew the curtain around the
bed, hoping to block them out. But not seeing them only

made their noise sound louder—hysterical laughter, bad dirty jokes told in grating tones. I wanted to scream at them to shut up, but for some reason I was afraid. I looked over at Jack. He was beginning to wake up. He wasn't moaning any more, but I knew he felt rotten.

"I'll tell them to be quiet," I said. Jack nodded his head. I stuck my head out from the curtains. "Listen, could you try to be a little quieter? Jack's just come out of a big operation and he feels pretty bad." There was immediate silence, and everyone stared at me.

"Sure," Mike said. "I'm sorry. We'll keep it down."

I waited for the silence to turn into quiet whispers. I didn't just hate them for their noise and background. I hated them for their health.

jack

When I awoke, the euphoria had worn off and I ached all over. They gave me a shot, which helped a little but not much. I felt as though I'd just fought ten rounds with Muhammad Ali. I was aware of a dull ache in my hip where they had taken the bone fragment which was now fused in my neck. I had a terrible, raspy sore throat where they'd placed a tube during the operation, and it hurt me to swallow or even talk. I also felt terribly nauseated.

I thought Joe had said that the nausea was caused by the morphine. When the evening nurse came to give me another morphine shot, I was dubious and told her what Joe had said. She explained that the nausea was caused by the anesthetic and gave me the shot. It killed the pain.

The next few days were awful. I felt that up to the time of the operation I was beginning to make progress, but that now I was so sick and sore I couldn't stand it. It felt like a real setback, which depressed me, which in turn depressed Mary. Joe said that by Sunday I would feel better. And on Sunday I did feel better, at least well enough to start thinking once again about the future. Now that the fusion was successful Mary and I both wanted to know how much longer I'd have to be in traction and when we could look forward to going to the Rusk Institute for rehabilitation.

"We better get these strong because you're going to need them," Janet said. I was lying on my stomach, and she was massaging my shoulders, arms, and fingers and talking to me about what rehabilitation would be like. "Even if you've got only one leg, they can get you up and walking," she said. "But you can't get impatient. It takes a baby ten months to begin to walk and then a couple of more months before it learns how to keep its balance. You're in exactly the same position, and you may need braces and crutches at first. It'll probably take the same amount of time, and you're probably going to need your arms to push yourself around in a wheelchair and your shoulders to carry you on crutches when they get you on your feet. It'll be harder than anything you've ever done, Jack."

I didn't think so. It couldn't be harder than lying here and waiting for return. I thought again about movies I'd seen of guys in wheelchairs getting up between parallel bars, pulling themselves along, learning how to walk. That was exercise and work, but at least I'd be helping myself. I was exercising now, but there weren't many muscles to exercise—only those few in my left leg. The rest of the time was still spent lying there and hoping other muscles would return.

Janet was always telling me to push like hell to get to Rusk. "We've done about all we can for you to get you medically healthy," she said. "You'll have to push to get out of here because sometimes we can get possessive."

"Joe's not like that," I said.

"No, he's not. But you still must push hard. I'll help you."

When I asked Joe how much longer he thought I'd have to stay in Southampton, he said four weeks. "Just as soon as I'm sure the fusion has taken and that they've got a bed for you at Rusk."

The waiting became interminable. The days were long and boring. Now that the danger was past and we thought I'd walk again, Mary finally began to let down and the strain began to show. She looked tired and drawn and began to worry about details, especially money. Blue Cross and Blue Shield paid for my hospital and part, but only a small part, of the doctors' bills. We already owed $5000 and were told that the Rusk Institute would cost about $1000 a week and wasn't covered by Blue Cross. I tried to assure her that it would be okay, that only we mattered, and that we had the rest of our lives to pay off our debts. I wasn't putting on an act just to make her feel better—I really wasn't concerned about money. I had seen death—total paralysis. I had touched bottom. But now I was on my way up again. I didn't know how far I could go, nor could I imagine how hard it would be to return to a somewhat "normal" life. But getting there was the only thing that mattered. I couldn't worry about things like money. I could always borrow. Friends and family had already come forward and offered to help us. I'd worry about paying it back when I was on my feet.

I convinced Mary to spend more time at the beach and to nap instead of coming to be with me at dinnertime. But I was hardly ever alone. If she didn't come herself, she always made sure one of the family, hers or mine, was with me.

The physical therapist I had wasn't working out. He seemed content to take me through a range of motion exercises. He never gave me a real workout. Mary and I began working together on the sly. I showed her how to give me the resistance exercises Joe had taught me. Every day we worked for half an hour on our own. She resisted with her thin body while I pushed and pulled my arms and wrists, left leg and ankle, against her weight.

The exercises did a lot for me; physically they gave me some small sense of well-being. And we saw improvements. Each day I'd be a little stronger than the day before, until one day I'd do something remarkable like let my leg dangle off the side of the frame and then lift it up again by myself. Or I would lie on my stomach and bend my left leg up at the knee nine or maybe ten times.

We'd work to the point of exhaustion. Lifting my leg nine or ten times gave me the same sense of mental and physical well-being that jogging a mile had before. I was again enjoying a sense of physicality. I was no longer just an object people did things for and to. Now I could begin to help myself through exercise. I began to get a better image of myself and when I exercised fought off the boredom and depression.

One day I suddenly wiggled the toes in my right foot, though the movement was very slight. Then I lost the connection, and for two days I couldn't move them at all. I began to lose confidence and even doubted that I'd ever moved them. But Joe said it was possible that I'd lost contact only temporarily with the nerves and in time would be able to move the foot again.

I spent all my spare time concentrating on those toes, thinking about them, trying to find the nerve circuitry that led to the muscle that could make them move. Slowly I found the nerves and began to gain control over them. I could now wiggle them on command but soon realized that that was all I could do with the right foot.

I was worried but tried not to show it to Mary. The first thing I did every morning was demonstrate to her how much stronger the left leg was getting. There was always a new trick—I'd push against her hand or pull up against her or wiggle my right toes hello. Then one day she picked up my right leg and bent it at the knee. I began pushing it out, the way I had the left leg, and it suddenly straightened out. I had to ask her to be sure. "Did my leg straighten out?"

"Yes," she said.

"Did I do it?"

"You must have. I didn't."

I wanted to try it again immediately to make sure I had done it. I couldn't feel the actual movement, but I was able to straighten the leg again. When Joe came in on rounds, he began playing with my left leg. Then he picked up the right. "Wiggle the toes," he ordered.

"Forget that," I said. "Pick up my leg and bend it at the knee—one hand on my heel and one behind my knee."

He looked at me, started to say something, didn't, and then did what I said.

"Watch," I said and straightened out my leg. Joe got a

funny look on his face—the same look Mike had described when I first moved my left leg. He tried other things with my right leg. All of a sudden I had movement in the ankle and calf. "It's there, Joe. I can feel it."

"Thanks for telling me," he said as he kept working my legs. Then he came around to the side of the bed and grabbed my hands. He told me to move my fingers, but I couldn't. There was nothing there. I heard him mumble something, more to himself than to me. "I can't believe they're not going to come back soon," he said.

"What makes you so sure?" I asked.

"I'm not, except that it looks as if you might get it all back."

I realized that was an incredible statement for him to make, but it didn't really excite me. I was now so used to waiting. Also, my hands were last on my personal priority list. I was already teaching myself to pinch by manipulating my wrist. Even if there was no return in my hands, surgery could help. Joe could transfer tendons from my elbows or wrist to my fingers, giving me at least partial use of my hands. What I cared most about now was sex and my legs.

I wondered about my leg. Had the nerves just suddenly healed or had they been there for some time without my knowing it? Had I just discovered them? Were there other nerves in my body that were okay? Were there muscles that I could be using that I wasn't—if so, would I have to rediscover every nerve circuit and relearn every movement? Everything I did, every move I made would be a first time. And that meant that I not only had to discover the correct circuitry to move a muscle; I also had to repeat it constantly to establish it firmly in my body's memory again. I was getting some idea of how "return" worked. Wiggling the toes on my left foot was already second nature. I didn't really have to think about it, and, of course, the more I moved the toes, the stronger the muscles got.

Often the muscles tired early, so that even though I'd established a pattern of movement, I couldn't always keep it up.

I was like a weight lifter who after five lifts can't even budge the weight. Except that I was lifting the weight of only part of my own body—a toe, a foot. I was getting an insight into the real meaning of the phrase "to be as weak as a baby."

One morning my legs spasmed. I got a terrible cramp as they contorted. I asked Mike to call for a nurse to straighten my legs out. He rang but there was no response, so he began calling for someone. I was getting more cramps. I began to try to move my legs myself. All of a sudden I did it. I lifted my left leg up in the air and bent it at the knee at the same time. Then I moved it to the left and straightened it out and set it down.

I got so excited that I practiced until my leg was too tired to move. If I can do this, I can walk, I thought, because all walking is is picking up your leg and putting it down. After the lights were out, I tried to move my left leg again, and I found I could lift it up, bend the knee, and put it down again. I wondered how long it had been there without my knowing it. What if I hadn't had the spasm and been uncomfortable? Maybe it would have been weeks before I would have discovered it and started using that muscle.

This new discovery made me even more anxious to get out of the hospital and into Rusk. I wanted to find out what muscles I did have. There was no way for me to know the extent of nerve damage to my abdomen, back, or internal organs while I was still in traction and catheterized. I did know I had my hips, however. One day when Mary and I were talking and I was lying on my stomach I decided to experiment and see if I could hump the bed. My movements were crude, my rhythm was off, and I tired quickly. But we were both elated with the promise of what that meant. "That's it," Mary said excitedly. "Looks pretty sexy to me." A nurse stuck her head in the door and said, "If I were you, I'd take the catheter out first, Mr. Willis." That night I ran my hands under the sheet to my groin and felt where they had shaved my pubic hair. I then ran my fingers up along my body. It was the first time I had done that since the accident. I didn't know why I was doing it, but suddenly I realized I felt a sense of wholeness. For the first time in six weeks I somehow had a sense of my entire body. I felt connected from head to toe. I was no longer a lot of disparate parts. I felt like a person.

I didn't know whether that feeling was the result of some final nerve connection that rendered me "whole" or whether I had been capable of feeling that way for a while and had just discovered it. But I ran my hands up and down my body in wonder.

With the feeling of wholeness came another phenomenon. The spasticity that had occurred only in my feet and legs now racked and jerked my entire body. It seemed to begin in my lower back and extend downward through my hips and legs to my feet. I would be lying perfectly still and suddenly my entire body would spasm. I might suddenly jerk and the lower part of my body would kick or lift off the bed, or I would suddenly tense up and straighten out as if somewhere inside me were a coiled steel spring that was being pulled from opposite ends of my body.

One day while Ann was bathing me, I suddenly spasmed, my leg flew up, and I kicked her in the back of the head. She didn't know what had happened. But Clive was standing behind her, so she swore at him for hitting her. I broke up.

For the first time being in traction became a nuisance. As

long as I was paralyzed it didn't bother me because I never felt motivated to move. I just didn't feel like going anywhere. Nor did I get uncomfortable if I lay in one position for a long time. But now, lying in traction, fastened by the tongs, became hell. I ached from lying in one position, and I couldn't move to alleviate the pain. And worst of all, I now *wanted* to move, to get up, to go somewhere, and I couldn't.

It seemed an incredible paradox—the better I got the worse I felt, the more I was subject to fits of depression, the more I felt trapped by my environment. I tried sleeping more—something I used to do in college when I was depressed. But when I awoke I still felt tied down and trapped. I remembered a picture of Gulliver tied down by thousands of tiny ropes, his arms at his sides, his neck stretched out. That's how I felt.

I became more sensitive to the moods of the nurses and aides. One day there seemed to be something tense and frantic in the air. I knew something had happened but didn't know what. When my brother came to visit me, he said he had just bumped into Joe.

"There was another accident," he said.

"What happened?"

"Some guy, twenty-two, was tossed by a wave. He's paralyzed from the shoulders down."

"Where's he now?" I said.

"I don't know. That's all Joe said. He looked very tired."

When the nurses came in, I asked them about the kid, but they said they didn't know anything about him except that he was now on the operating table. Around three in the morning one of the nurses told me that the boy was out of surgery but was in pretty bad shape. He'd fractured the two vertebrae higher than the ones I'd broken. The higher the fracture and injury to the cord, the more extensive the damage and less likely the possibility of recovery.

Joe looked exhausted when he came in the next morning. "How's the kid?" I asked.

"Pretty bad. He's going to need a lot of help. Maybe you can talk with him in a couple of weeks."

"Sure, I'd be happy to." But I wondered what I could say to him except to wait and see what happened.

I couldn't put him out of my mind. I'd never met him, but I was getting progressively depressed thinking about him. It was tough enough to be thirty-six years old and have to face paralysis, but to be in your early twenties and have that happen seemed impossible to me. I remembered how confused I'd been at that age, in school, worrying about the army and what to do with my life. I couldn't imagine having to face all those problems and be paralyzed on top of it.

Thinking about him made me think about myself. I thought I was getting better, and I thought I knew what I wanted out of life. But deep down I wasn't any more prepared to face paralysis than he was. And now that I was beginning to get movement, I wanted to cry when I thought of what was ahead of him.

mary

I walked slowly down the hall. It was early afternoon, and everyone, including Jack, seemed to be dozing. I stopped outside the room of the young man who'd broken his neck. Everyone spoke about him in hushed tones, and until this moment I hadn't really thought about him. They all said he was in very bad shape, that he was paralyzed from his neck down and would never get better because he'd severed his cord. How did they know, I'd asked one of the nurses who had watched him being operated on. "You could see the spinal fluid spilling out all over the place," was the answer.

I stared into the room, which looked dark and airless. I could hardly see his face, but I could tell that his eyes were open. He could still blink his eyes. I wondered what he was thinking as he lay there, totally motionless. He had a short, dumpy body, and I noticed that his feet, soft and swollen, were wrapped in pieces of the same furry sheepskin he was lying on. They looked just like pigs-in-a-blanket.

The next morning I saw the boy's mother in his room. She was a squat woman with a warm face, who was wearing a matronly cotton-print dress that accentuated her large, soft bosom. I wasn't sure of her nationality, but she looked Italian. I watched her fuss around her son. She straightened and dusted and adjusted every object in the room. I could see exactly how she was in her own house. She had transformed the impersonal Southampton hospital room into "the sick room" merely by her presence. I could see that she occasionally asked her son questions that he seemed to ignore.

One afternoon we literally bumped into each other in the tiny Surgical One kitchen, where I stored the fruit Jell-O Libbie made for Jack. The woman was cooking soup for her son. She turned toward me, a smile on her face. "He just won't eat anything," she said with gentle exasperation. "I've tried as many of his favorite things as I can . . . but he's so

depressed." She paused. "I hear your husband is doing well.
Maybe it will be the same with my boy."

"I hope so," I said and left the kitchen. I wanted to get
away from her. I didn't ask her how her son was feeling. I
didn't try to draw her out about how she was feeling. I was
just beginning to believe that Jack was getting better, that we
were both moving ahead, slowly, very slowly, but moving. I
didn't want to be weighed down in any way by someone
else's sorrow. I didn't want to be lumped together with "the
families of quadriplegics." A few days later she came over to
me to say she'd heard that Jack was going to the Rusk Institute.

"Oh, I hope Jimmy can go there . . . but Mrs. LaVinio
says it's very expensive. I also heard the waiting list's very
long and you need connections." She looked up at me and
smiled, her eyes not quite pleading, but placating. "I know
your father's a doctor," she said. "And I thought maybe he
could help us."

I felt my back go up. "His connection isn't direct," I said.
"We'll help if we can, but . . ." She put her arm out and pat-
ted my wrist.

"I just heard they can do such amazing things with them.
Can teach them how to feed and care for themselves."

I didn't know how to get away from her, from a discussion
that was making me so uncomfortable I felt sick. I just stood
there, looking down at this kind-faced woman, feeling four
times her height yet dwarfed by her persistence. I really
wanted to remind her how much better off Jack was than
her son, that they weren't the same at all. All I heard was,
"They can do such wonderful things with *them*." Why
couldn't I have simply said, "Sure, we'll help you if we can,"
and left it at that?

I walked back to Jack's room, trying to figure out why the
short discussion with her had upset me. I knew I had been

coldhearted, and I felt guilty. Why couldn't I even allow myself to feel sorry for her, to empathize, to help? Maybe it was because I couldn't think of Jack as a cripple, as one of "them."

The next morning when I came in, Jack looked sad and depressed. I knew he was recovering quickly from the operation, that he'd been feeling better the night before.

"What's the matter?" I said. "You look terrible."

"That kid died late last night. He's dead."

I was shocked. Dead. How could he be dead? "What happened?"

Jack stared straight ahead. "He must have developed pneumonia very quickly. They did a tracheotomy on him to help him breathe, but it got worse. The nurses were running back and forth all night. Joe came in and tried to save him. But there was nothing they could do. He died around midnight."

"I don't believe it," I said dumbly. "His mother seemed so optimistic yesterday. She asked me to help them get him into Rusk. Was she here when he died?"

"I don't know," Jack said.

"Maybe it's better . . . I don't know. They knew he'd severed his cord."

"How can it be better when a twenty-two-year-old kid dies like that?"

"I didn't mean that," I said defensively. "I just meant . . ."

"I'm sorry." Jack looked sympathetically at me. "It's just really upset me—more than I would have thought."

I was thinking about the mother. I wondered where she was. Before I left the hospital that night, I walked past his room. The boy's death seemed real only when I saw his empty bed and realized that his mother was no longer there.

jack

"Hey, someone wake Mike up."

About ten nurses and aides had come into the room. One of them shook Mike, who was taking his prelunch snooze.

"C'mon, Mike, wake up. Wall Street needs you," Clive said. Mike had been a clerk on Wall Street before he got hurt.

"Hey, what's going on?" he said, ignoring Clive.

Paper cups were passed around, and the nurses were all giggly as Janet brought in the Champale. The cork popped and the bottle was poured. "Happy birthday, Mike," someone said, and we all sang "Happy Birthday" to him and sipped our drinks from paper cups.

"Hey, Jack, hey, man, we should do this every day," Mike hollered. "All we need now is some dope."

"You're dope enough for us," someone said.

We toasted Mike's arm and leg, his girl friend, Muggs, my big toe, the hamstring in my left leg, the nurses and aides. Then Mike made a special toast to a nurse's aide we called "Hands" because she gave the best massages in the hospital. An aide with the most beautiful black skin saw that I was sweating. She came over and wiped my forehead. "Not used to partying, honey?"

"I guess not."

She pulled back my sheet and rubbed talcum powder on my shoulders and chest. Then when she was sure nobody was watching she quickly pulled the sheet all the way down and with a twinkle in her eye sprinkled powder all over my balls. I grinned and swooned. Mike saw what she had done. "Hey, it's my birthday," he said. "Not his."

Janet ordered the rest of the nurses back to work, warning them not to mention our party to anyone.

Mike was improving rapidly. His doctors had finally removed the cast from his arm. With his arm out of traction, he was now able to get up out of bed and into a wheelchair for an hour or so each day.

I watched as he sat on the edge of the bed, apprehensive and dizzy. Janet would help lift him onto his feet, where he'd stand briefly and then pirouette into the chair. He was much stronger than I was, yet the struggle into the chair was tremendous, and he got very uncomfortable and dizzy the first few times he tried to get up. I wondered how it would be for me.

Scotty, a night nurse, told me of a paraplegic they'd had in Southampton several years before. He said that when this guy got to Rusk, he had a great deal of difficulty adjusting to the place. One day they just dumped him onto the floor in a room with nothing but his wheelchair and told him that he'd have to stay there unless he could lift himself into the chair. I didn't know if the story was true. But I did know that the Rusk Institute was tough. I'd heard plenty of stories about it. Howard Rusk was an old army doctor, and a public relations man who was supposed to run the place very much like an army hospital. Nobody was babied, and just as soon as possible you were forced to get dressed and up into a wheelchair to begin exercises. But it was supposed to be the best, and I just wanted to get there. I knew I could handle it, and the sooner I got up and could start helping myself the better off I'd be. But I was also afraid of what I might find out about myself. Would my back support me? Could I walk without braces? How whole would I be?

In spite of my fears, I was ready to get out of Southampton and to start rehabilitation. Janet also thought I was ready. But for some reason Joe kept putting off the decision. At first, right after the operation, he'd said it would be four weeks, but now two weeks were up and he'd still said nothing about when I might leave, even though he knew how anxious I was to get back to New York.

The days dragged as we waited. I was bored and getting more irritable. Little things continued to annoy Mary. We had a small problem with our apartment. All it meant was a call to our landlord, but when he was nasty with her, she got terribly upset. Money, too, continued to worry her, in spite of my assurances that it was going to be okay. She was looking more and more tired and depressed. The tension of being constantly with me, of handling our financial affairs, of dealing with doctors, families, and friends, was just too much. Her easy laughter didn't come often any more. She began to get away in the afternoons, to spend more time at the beach. While this was what I wanted, it made things more difficult for me. Without her, the days went even slower.

I was still immobilized in traction and couldn't read unless I was on my stomach. So I spent whole hours alone, just staring at the ceiling or kibitzing with Mike, even though now he spent more and more time outside in his wheelchair. I wanted more than anything else to get out, to get up and be with Mary, to have a family, to go back to work.

Friends asked me if I thought about living my life differently now. To my amazement, I realized that I didn't want to do anything differently; I just wanted to get back to where I was. I knew people tried to make trade-offs, like "Please, God, just let me walk and I'll be a better person." Baloney. If I'd thought it would help, I would have bargained. But, first of all, I didn't believe it would work, and even if it did, I knew I could never live up to my end of the bargain. So I'd lose either way. It would be just my luck. I'd promise to be good, and the first time I screwed up, which would probably be my first day out of the hospital, I'd have to worry about getting hit by lightning.

But others were praying for me. Janet told me she said daily prayers for me. And one morning a priest came in to visit Mike. He was short, wore glasses, and though he looked about my age, was almost completely bald. He had to go around me to get to Mike, so he stopped to say hello and asked me what had happened to me. I told him, and he told me that his name was Father Vitalis. I thought he was kidding, but he was a very serious man who spoke in a soft Slavic voice. Before he left, he asked if I'd mind if he said a blessing for me. I didn't mind, and he made the sign of the cross, folded his hands on my bed, closed his eyes, and prayed for my recovery in the name of The Father, The Son, and The Holy Ghost. A few days later when he came in, he said, "What religion are you?" I told him I was a Jewish atheist.

"Impossible," he said. "You can't be Jewish and an atheist." We argued religion for a while, and before he left he asked again if he could say a blessing for me. I said, "Please," and he crossed himself again and began to pray, "In the name of Abraham and Isaac . . ."

Father Vitalis stopped by often after that. It didn't seem to bother him or Janet that I didn't believe in God. I realized that if their faith was the source of their strength, I was too grateful for that to care where it came from. I looked forward to their visits and prayers as much as I welcomed the warmth of friends who either visited or took the time to write me.

We must have gotten between five and ten letters a day, and on weekends the room was always crowded with friends. I wondered what effect I'd had on the lives of people who wrote to me. A friend of Mary's said, "Your friends become spectators in a situation like this, but that shouldn't disqualify them from cheering you on." A woman from the office whom I hardly knew sent me cards every week. I tried to remember if I'd ever been particularly nice to her. I wondered if she understood what my life might be like. I made a mental note to ask her when I got out of the hospital. In a way it was like being at one's own funeral and hearing the eulogy and praise of all those who knew and cared for you.

mary

The beaches emptied after Labor Day. A steady stream of cars, piled high with bicycles, boxes, barbecues, and beach gear, had lined the Montauk Highway from Sunday night straight through to Wednesday. Long Island belonged once again to the locals and to a few hangers-on.

Janet LaVinio had been urging us to leave, to get Jack started with his rehabilitation as soon as possible, but Joe was more conservative. "Just want to make sure that fusion is taking," he said. But we'd received word from the Rusk Institute that a bed would be ready by September 15, and my family was already making plans to leave. Papa and my sister, Annie, would go the week before, and my mother and I would close the house.

Libbie had wanted to stay until we left, but we convinced her that she was needed more in Los Angeles, where Lou had been alone for a month. There was a tearful good-bye, mixed with relief on both sides. We were all going home. . . .

My mother and I hung out clean, damp towels on a clothesline. The potatoes had been harvested, and the fields were dusty and dry. One strong breeze and everything was covered with dust. Looking now at those flat, dry fields, it was hard to imagine that they had been green with fat potato plants most of the summer and would be green and fat again.

"Where do you think you'll live when we get back to New York?" my mother asked.

"Live? What do you mean? I'll stay in the apartment." I really didn't understand what she was asking.

"But whose apartment? Yours and Jack's or home?"

Now I understood. There was "home," and there was Jack's and my apartment—and the two were not one and the same, at least not in Mama's eyes.

"I'll live in Jack's and my apartment. Why?"

"I just thought it would be easier for you if you lived with us," my mother said. "You won't have to worry about cooking or keeping house. . . . I just thought it would be nicer, that's all."

For a moment the idea appealed to me, but then I thought about "going back home" to live and realized I didn't want to do that at all. Living alone in our apartment both frightened and appealed to me. It would be physically easier with my parents, but physical comfort didn't seem as important to me as privacy—just being alone with myself.

"No, Mama. All my things are in our apartment. I really feel that's home. I know it may be difficult, but I'm not too worried. I even look forward to being there."

My mother looked concerned and disappointed. "All right, darling. But you can always change your mind."

I waited a moment outside Jack's room. Clive stood near him and poured a large glob of white lotion on his back. I watched his huge, strong hands work the liquid into Jack's back, slowly and evenly. Jack's ribs showed through his skin, which looked especially pale next to Clive's black hands and forearms. Clive rubbed more lotion into Jack's legs, which were so thin that I was sure Clive could have wrapped his whole hand around the thigh. I watched him lift Jack's leg and bend it at the knee, gently bouncing it back and forth toward Jack's back. The muscle was so tight that I could see it twitch under the smooth skin of Jack's knee.

"Got to keep those muscles loose," Clive said. "Okay, Jack. You bring that leg up without me."

The hamstring muscle began to strain like the taut string of a bow. Clive looked on patiently, excitement and real pride filling his eyes. Jack's leg started to fall to one side.

"Come on, you can do it. Just keep it comin'," Clive said.

Jack struggled silently to keep the leg from falling. Once

past the halfway mark, he was all right. I thought I saw the muscles in his lower back begin to share the burden of the leg's weight. He did it. The leg swayed a little but stayed at a firm right angle, the toes pointing toward the ceiling. It seemed so little, but I felt tremendously excited. Jack heard me come into the room.

"I can do a new trick," he said proudly.

"I know. I saw it. I was standing outside. It's fabulous."

I bent down and kissed Jack's shoulder, which was still slippery and sweet with body lotion. Clive was immediately more formal with me in the room. In a way, I wished I'd stayed outside longer. There was a bond of love and unarticulated loyalty between them, the kind of friendship I imagined men share when they're fighting a war together.

"Guess I'd better get you over on your back," Clive said, a smile curling his lips. "Then you two can be more loving." And he broke into an embarrassed giggle. He placed the sheepskins on Jack's back, easily lifted and placed the frame on top of the sheepskins, quickly strapped Jack in tight, and with enormous grace and ease turned the whole contraption over without the slightest bump or jolt.

Lying on his back, Jack let his left leg hang over the edge of the bed. "Watch this, Mary," he said and began to swing his leg back and forth, building up momentum with each swing. Then with one big heave and sigh, he let the leg fall back onto the bed.

"When did you discover you could do that?" I said excitedly.

"I've been working on it," Jack said. "I've started to try it with the right, but it's still too weak."

"Let me see it again." As I watched him swing his leg like the weighty pendulum of a big clock, I realized I'd never seen him move so dramatically. Whenever I spoke to Joe or asked him questions, I always saw how far Jack still had to go, and I always felt depressed and exhausted thinking about it. Joe could never tell me simply what I wanted to hear—that Jack would walk.

"We still don't know if he has back muscles or how strong his hips are," was Joe's guarded professional response.

But watching Jack now, I didn't think about all the muscles he might not have. I saw movement, real muscle action. When I helped him do his exercises and felt him push against my arm, I felt real pressure, the twinges and jerks of muscles. His legs were alive, and at times like this I felt as though they'd never been dead, never lain on those clean, white hospital sheets like logs, like a lot of dead wood.

I felt real pride in Jack's physical accomplishments and liked him to show off for friends. I didn't realize that part of my motivation was to *prove* to the world that Jack was going to be all right, that *my* man wasn't a cripple. His infirmity reflected on me in ways so subtle that I was unaware of their effect. I only knew that as anxious as I was to leave Southampton, I was also very scared about resuming a life in New York. Showing people what Jack could do was a way of warning them, warning myself, of the difficulties that lay ahead and of our desire to conquer them.

jack

The harder I pushed Joe to set a firm date, the more stubborn he seemed to get. Finally one morning I apologized for pushing him and said I'd leave it up to him. That tack worked, as I'd known it would, and he said he understood my anxiety. Two days later he told me I could be moved the Monday after Labor Day. That night I worried that maybe he was just committing himself to a day to satisfy me and perhaps it was really too early for me to move.

I panicked a little. What if I wasn't really ready to be moved? Suppose they took me out of traction too early and I hurt my spine? I should have been laughing at myself. For three weeks I had pushed Joe to commit himself to a date and let me out of the hospital. Now that he had set the date, I was scared *he* was making a mistake. I should have laughed, but I couldn't because I was too scared.

It was Friday, three days before I was to be moved to Rusk. Joe held a small screwdriver in his hand. "This is the day," he said. "How'd you like to sit up?" He began unscrewing the toggle bolts in my head. I didn't feel any pain. One side came loose, then the other. I felt him remove the tongs from my head and sensed rather than felt that the weights, too, had been removed.

"Don't move," Joe ordered. "Don't move your head."

Janet handed him the neck brace I had been outfitted for two weeks earlier. Joe slowly and very slightly lifted my head and slid part of the brace behind my neck. Then he gently laid my head back and fitted the front part under my chin and strapped the back and front together.

"How does that feel?" he asked.

"Okay, I guess. Maybe a little loose."

He made a couple of adjustments. "How about now?"

"Better."

I still hadn't lifted my head. But I could tell that with my chin held high and the back of my head supported and pushed a bit forward, my movement would be limited.

"Okay," Joe said, "get him into bed."

There was some scurrying while some of the nurses went searching for an empty bed. Clive pushed my frame into the hall and placed it near the regular hospital bed. Janet carefully carried the pole and drainage bag to which my catheter was attached. There was a brief conference about how to transfer me from the frame to the bed. Then Clive and three nurses grabbed the sheepskins on one side while Joe held my head and pulled me, sheepskins and all, onto the bed.

I felt funny in the bed. It was so soft after nine weeks in the frame, and I was so used to being forced to stare at the ceiling that I hadn't moved a muscle.

"Smile," Joe said. "You're out of traction." Everyone stood around me and grinned proudly, and I felt as if I'd just been bar mitzvahed. Then they wheeled me back inside the room.

Joe pulled up the sides of the crib-like bed so I wouldn't roll off. He tested the bars to make sure they were secure.

"Can I sit up?"

"In a while," he said.

"Can I roll over?"

"Anything. Just take it easy."

"Does Mary know?"

"No." Janet smiled.

I gingerly tried to roll onto my left side, but couldn't do it. The neck brace was a little awkward, and without wrenching myself over, I didn't have enough strength to do it easily. With my left arm I reached out and grabbed a bar on the upraised side of the bed and slowly pulled myself over onto my left side and rested my head on the pillow. I looked up and found myself staring directly into Mike's eyes. For what was probably ten seconds but seemed like ten minutes, we silently stared at each other as if we were trying to be sure we were really the same two people who had shared that room for nine weeks. We were like two blind men who have been brought together and can now suddenly see. I broke the silence first.

"Jesus. Are you thin!"

"You look worse," Mike said. "We both look like we just came out of a Japanese prison camp."

We laughed together, but I was shocked. If I looked worse than Mike, I knew I was in bad shape, worse than I'd imagined. Suddenly I realized I hadn't seen my own face since the morning of the accident. I felt frail and weak, like a tiny wounded animal in that crib of a bed. I asked Mike to ring for Janet.

"How much do you think I weigh?" I asked her.

She looked at my body, put her arm underneath my hips and lifted me just a little. "Maybe a hundred and twenty-five pounds," she said.

"I don't believe it. I couldn't have lost forty pounds. I bet I weigh less than Mary."

"Well, maybe you weigh a hundred and thirty pounds," she said, trying to make me feel a little better.

"Janet. Let me try to sit up."

"Okay. But not too far. We don't want you passing out."

She went down to the end of the bed and slowly began to crank me up. I tensed, expecting to get dizzy or feel nauseated. At about a thirty-three-degree angle, she stopped. "How do you feel?" she said.

"Fine. I think I could go higher."

But she left me there, more reclining than sitting. It felt good to be "up." The neck brace weighed heavily on me and didn't seem to fit quite right, but I hardly noticed it as I looked around at the room I'd never really seen. From my new vantage point, it seemed even smaller and dingier than I'd thought it was. I wondered how the Willises and Pleshettes and especially Mary had been able to come to this room day after day to be with me. From my bed I could now see the bright sunlight through the window and without too much trouble imagine what it felt like to be out in the hot sun, lazing in the sand or jogging along the beach. I tortured myself with those memories until Mary came in.

I was struck again by how thin and tired she looked. Her face was drawn, and most of her tan was gone. Her breasts were almost nonexistent under her shift. But she still looked lovely to me. Her face lit up when she saw me as she practically ran into the room to hug me. I grinned. "Baby. It's so nice to see you at eye level again."

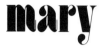

"The tongs. They took the tongs out," I said, looking straight and level and incredulously into Jack's eyes.

"Well, what do you think?"

"I think . . . I can't believe you're actually sitting up without those meat hooks in your head."

Jack was smiling and opened his arms to embrace me. He was wearing a neck brace and was so thin that he looked lost in the regular-size bed.

"I won't break," he said as I gingerly hugged him. "It's okay, doll. You won't hurt me."

I felt as though I were hugging a young boy. I could feel his bones. His chest was narrow, almost concave. I closed my eyes and gently passed my hands over his angular shoulders, down his skinny arms. His body felt unfamiliar.

"I'm skin and bones, aren't I?" Jack said. "They let me look at myself in the mirror and I hardly recognized myself."

I burst into tears, overwhelmed by this strange new physical closeness. I was sitting near Jack on the bed, feeling his body near mine for the first time in two months, and I was both happy and horrified.

"It's not that bad, is it?" Jack said, laughing, smoothing my hair with his tightly fisted hand.

I tried to bury my head in his shoulder, but the neck brace got in the way. Then I took a deep breath and smiled back at Jack. "I'm just not used to seeing you face to face, that's all. It's so good not to have to look down at you, so good to touch you. I'll be all right. Just give me a few minutes to get used to you." I got up and walked to the foot of the bed to see Jack from a short distance. Then I walked around the bed to see him from all sides. "I guess you *are* pretty skinny," I said. "You look like the ninety-eight-pound weakling who gets sand kicked in his face."

Mike started to laugh, and before I knew it we were all laughing.

I lay awake listening to the chirps and creaks of the country. I saw Jack's long, thin, pale face—not the face of memories, not even the face I'd grown accustomed to staring down at for nine weeks. I hadn't realized how much weight he'd lost. When he was flat on his back, he'd looked fatter, maybe because the weight of him spread him out a little, the way my thighs always look fatter when I'm sitting or lying down.

I thought about Jack's description of the silent moment when he and Mike first looked at each other. And then it really hit me that these two men who'd been sharing their room and their lives so intimately had never actually seen each other until that moment.

"I thought I really looked bad," Mike had said. "Then I got a look at him and I felt a little better."

There had been a hysterical quality to the laughing and joking, a need to overcome the shock of seeing Jack without being solemn or serious. But now, lying alone, I was haunted by Jack's thin face and sunken eyes. He looked terrible, really emaciated and weak; admitting that to myself made me feel guilty and afraid.

I wanted to run back to him right away. I wanted to get used to him so I could feel attracted to him again. That's what was upsetting me. I wasn't attracted to this shrunken-looking man. All my worrying about sex seemed at this moment an intellectual dilemma, an exercise of the brain because I felt nothing of my body, not a jot of passion. It was as though all sex had been squeezed out of me, and Jack's thinness and physical weakness only seemed to confirm my dried-out feeling of sexlessness.

I closed my eyes tightly. "Oh, please, let everything be

okay," I prayed out loud. "Let everything work out and be happy and normal again." And then I reiterated my ritual list of wishes, the way most people count sheep, and tried to fall asleep.

Mary and her mother arrived early with a box of little gifts for the hospital staff. We were going back to New York. As usual Clive fed, bathed, shaved me, and brushed my teeth. But this was the last time. It felt like graduation day.

Joe had come in earlier to say good-bye. "Good luck," he said. "Come back to see us."

"Thanks, Joe. Thanks for everything."

"I think you're going to be okay," he said as he left the room.

Now the room was packed with nurses and aides who had come to say good-bye. Some had even come in on their day off. There was lots of kissing and hugging as all of us nervously killed time, waiting for the ambulance to arrive.

"I told you he'd get out of this place before me," I heard Mike say.

"What do you expect?" one of the nurses quipped. "We can't lose both our dreamboats at the same time."

"Anyway," I said, "you'll get twice as much attention now with me gone."

"Whad'ya mean, twice as much?" Mike said. "I was getting that when you were here."

Everyone laughed. The room was crowded with white and pink uniforms. A seventeen-year-old aide quietly came over to my bed to say good-bye. "It's been great knowing you," she said, and blushed when I pulled her over and kissed her cheek.

"Hey. Can I do that when I leave?" Mike bellowed.

"Break it up, break it up," Janet LaVinio said as she sailed into the room. "Time for a little nursing." She pulled the sheet up, exposing my right buttock, and swiftly gave me a shot. "You're going to need a little morphine," she said. "It's a long drive in a neck brace. This will relax you." Then she turned on her heel. "Doesn't anyone have any work to do around here? Mrs. DiMaggio needs her bedpan emptied, and it's time for Mr. Simpson's pills."

The staff started to respond, but slowly. Everyone took his time leaving the room, each person coming up to say good-bye. "Stay in touch," they said. "We want to see you on your feet."

Janet came back into the room with two ambulance drivers. She showed them the bottle which was attached to my catheter and explained how they should maneuver with it. I was a little nervous that they might pull it too hard, but they seemed to understand what Janet was telling them. They were both young and strong, but Janet supervised their moving me from the bed to a rolling stretcher. One of them asked me if I was uncomfortable. "I'm okay. It just feels strange to be moving."

As they wheeled me out of the room, Janet tucked the rough gray wool ambulance blanket around my legs and waist. She smoothed my hair and ran her fingers around the neck brace to make sure I was comfortable. Her touch was a mother's touch. I glanced up and saw that Mary's mother was watching. There were tears in her eyes.

As they wheeled me down the hall, I could hear Mike complaining about the injustice of being left behind. Janet carried the pole with the bag attached to the catheter, and Clive helped Mary with our belongings. Outdoors, Janet gave me a kiss good-bye. Her eyes were smiling but moist. I looked up, saw the sky and breathed deeply, and then smiled up at Mary. Clive stood around awkwardly watching me. For the first time in nine weeks there was nothing for him to do. I grabbed his hand just before they lifted me into the ambulance.

"I'll miss you, Clive. Thank you."

He looked at me and pulled his hand away. Finally he